"My first impression was, "Wow what a journey!" But more importantly, I have never seen a more complete and simple guide to the development and growth of a hygienist. Any hygienists who can master these skills will forever be revered by all doctors they come in contact with."

K. Pat Brown, DDS

"I have had the privilege of working with Tiffany for the past five years, and I can tell you she is the real deal: a natural-born leader. She puts into practice what she preaches, and has an innate ability to get others to align with her goals. *Hygienepreneur* is more than just a title, it is a vision that Tiffany lives every day to achieve maximum success."

Matthew M. Wasemiller, DDS

"*Hygienepreneur* is the first book that encompasses the entire scope of being a successful hygienist. It provides helpful insight to scheduling, patient care considerations, and communication best practices—not just between my patients and me but also my front business team, and especially my doctor. I highly recommend this book to any hygienist who wants to become the **indispensable team member** and chart his/her own career path!"

Mary K. Hughes RDH, BS
Dental Entrepreneur Business Unit Leader

D1591087

"This book is truly inspiring as Tiffany shares her story of becoming not just a dental professional, but a "hygiene-preneuer." She brings her experience in customer service and business-building to the back office. She teaches you how to help your patient feel cared for and ultimately reach optimal health, while also helping the practice win. This book got me out of my day-to-day rut and inspired me to take action in my practice. I am now fulfilled in my career as a dental hygienist and excited to go to work and make a difference."

Alexandra Campbell, RDH, BS

"The practical, sound advice Tiffany presents will save you years of 'figuring it out.'" Scripts, protocols, sage advice...all the good stuff and more. Hygienepreneurs take control of their careers, their departments, and their lives. This book is Tiffany's roadmap for a win-win-win!"

Mike Czubiak, DDS

"This book has started a positive movement! The future of dental hygiene and the tools you need to truly uplift and support a dental office are all in this book. Hygienists everywhere will be energized and motivated to deliver the very best for their patients with less fatigue. The patient benefits and the practice soars!"

Cortney Dickert, RDH

"As a clinician, this book has helped me find the confidence I knew I always had!"

Nicole Gollhofer, RDH

"To the Dental community, this book is long overdue for the hard-working hygienists who strive to educate and care for their patients. Tiffany sees the opportunity to bring added value to the hygienist's professional life and, in turn, also adds value to the practice as a whole. I am excited to share Tiffany's book with my friends in the dental community!"

Kerri McCullough, Henry Schein Professional Practice Transitions

"This book is the real deal! Tiffany personally trained me using all of the tips that are discussed in the book. Working with her for the last three years has revolutionized the way I practice dental hygiene. Her main focus in the book is providing great patient care, and how to grow the dental practice. But there's so much more than that included! She is truly an advocate for the patient's dental health, and someone who naturally builds growth and production for the practice. Tiffany is the ultimate *Hygienepreneur,* and this book will be a huge eye-opener for the practice of dental hygiene everywhere!"

Shalon Ziegenhorn, RDH

"Tiffany has done an outstanding job of saying what EVERY doctor would love to say to the hygienists in their practice on how to be productive, proficient, efficient and effective in daily care for our patients. Five-star service delivered in a hygiene operatory that spreads like wildfire throughout the office CAN be achieved by following her system! Tiffany has a formula for a win-win-win experience which profits the patient, the hygienist, and the practice! You 'rock,' Tiffany, as a dental hygiene leader. Carry on and spread your positive message to your colleagues...their patients and doctors will be most appreciative!"

Terry L Watson, DMD

HYGIENEPRENEUR

HYGIENEPRENEUR

The Dental Hygienist's Guide to Achieving
Career Success & Personal Transformation

Tiffany Cavazos, RDH

ISBN: 978-0-678-90803-8

This book is dedicated to my amazing parents,
Mark and Rosemary Geiger.

Their example of extreme work ethic showed me how to hustle and survive in
any circumstance in life.

Thank you, Mom and Dad!

Contents

VI. THE FINAL FRONTIER: YOU

APPENDICES

INDEX

FOREWORD
Mark A. Costes, DDS

As far back as I can remember, I knew that I wanted to own my own business. Some of my oldest and fondest memories go back to long family dinners when my parents would tell stories of legendary relatives who had defied the odds, started with nothing more than simple ideas and hard work, and turned them into thriving businesses.

Those stories were the seeds that grew into a fascination with entrepreneurship and later led to my choice to become an entrepreneur. But even with that realization early in life, I didn't know exactly what that future would look like.

That all changed my junior year in high school during my very first varsity baseball game when I collided face-first with the left field fence after misjudging a home run that was hit in my direction.

The impact of the collision left me with several fractured and avulsed teeth as well as a broken jaw and multiple intra and extra-oral lacerations. The eighteen months that followed comprised an endless succession of appointments as a team of dentists and dental specialists worked together to restore the damage done to my mouth and face on the field on that fateful spring day.

Although it was a tedious and often painful process, the results were nothing short of miraculous. The dental team was not only gentle and kind, but they were also extremely skilled clinicians. I was in awe of their skill set, and from that experience forward I knew that I wanted to be able to help others in the same way that the team had helped me. I wanted to become a dentist.

Fortunately, dentistry, unlike other health-care professions, allows individuals who are interested in business ownership as well as the clinical practice of dentistry to flex their entrepreneurial muscle in many ways. And this is true for hygienists too!

Immediately after graduating from the Marquette University School of Dentistry in 2002, I went to work as an associate at a fast-paced private practice with the intention of improving my clinical speed and quality, while also learning more about the business side of running a dental practice. The owner-doctor was an incredible mentor, and he showed me the finer points of producing exceptional surgical and restorative outcomes in an efficient manner. Additionally, his office manager took me under her wing and taught me everything that I needed to know about the front office and practice management. It was the ideal real-life crash-course, and after just a year I felt confident enough to enter the world of dental-entrepreneurship.

I have been practicing dentistry for nineteen years and have owned a total of sixteen dental practices. But believe me, I don't say this to brag. In fact, I've probably made just about every mistake and bad decision possible during my journey. But what separated me from other struggling practice owners was the fact that I took every challenge and failure, learned from them, and carried on with stubborn persistence.

One of the overwhelming lessons that I've learned in practice ownership throughout my career is that **the hygiene department is the**

heart of any general dental practice. A thriving hygiene department can have a positive effect in all other areas of the practice, including doctor production and case acceptance; conversely, an anemic or dysfunctional hygiene department can lead to practices and practice owners that perpetually struggle.

I am honored that Tiffany has asked me to write the foreword for this book, but for me, it was an easy decision. The strategies and tactics covered in this book, if implemented, have the power to significantly up-level any hygiene department no matter where it falls on the spectrum.

From a doctor's perspective, Tiffany covers:

- How a hygiene department can "carry" the practice and decrease the burden that doctors often feel to make up for underperformance in hygiene.
- How to create a trickle-down effect that leads to improved practice culture which then leads to a happier, more productive team and an exceptional patient experience.
- How to create an atmosphere of positivity with less stress, drama, and chaos.

From a hygiene perspective, Tiffany discusses:

- How to deliver great service every time to create a "lifetime patient."
- How to structure a triple win-scenario for your patients, your practice and you.
- How to gain a feeling of "ownership" in your practice which leads to better clinical outcomes, better case acceptance, more production for the practice and a more rewarding and fulfilling career for the hygienist.

I truly believe that dentistry is the greatest profession on the planet, and I'm blessed to be a part of it. Whether you are a dentist, dental hygienist, or dental office manager, I wish you nothing but the best in your pursuit for a fulfilling career and a life with purpose.

Enjoy *HYGIENEPRENEUR!*

Committed to your success,

> ***Mark A. Costes, DDS***
> Founder, Dental Success Institute
> Co-founder, Dental Success Network
> Host, *Dentalpreneur* podcast
> #1 International best-selling author, *Pillars of Dental Success*

HYGIENEPRENEUR

The Dental Hygienist's Guide to Achieving
Career Success & Personal Transformation

INTRODUCTION
What Is a Hygienepreneur? (And How I Became One)

I'm Tiffany Cavazos and I'm a dental hygienist and consultant. I've written this book for one simple purpose: I want my fellow hygienists to be successful! I want you to become a *Hygienepreneur*.

So, what's a Hygienepreneur?

Simply put, it's a new type of hygienist—dynamic, entrepreneurial, and a breed apart. Utilizing a systematic method that I've developed, I train other hygienists in a proven approach to working within a dental practice to provide increased patient care and to increase production, while at the same time putting hygienists in charge of their own achievement. This repeatable, trainable program can enable you to help build a hygiene-centered dental practice that will help you, and the doctors you work with, drive growth and build success.

In the dental field, next to a career as a DDS or DMD, a career as a dental hygienist is the best position in terms of compensation, not to mention flexibility. Being a hygienist allows you to give your life beyond the workplace more time, while also allowing you to generate the income you need for a fulfilling life.

As a hygienist myself, I am in charge of the hygiene care my practice provides, and the success of its work, which has raised my professional and financial status. My numbers prove our success, and at our practice we are among an elite class of providers. My goal has always been to "produce" like a doctor does, and I am pleased to say that I have been doing this on a daily basis for many years now.

As the practice became successful, I frequently received many late-night and early-morning phone calls from other hygienists and dentists, who almost always wanted to ask me a quick question to help them solve a particular practice problem. The outcome of those calls was always the same: I would give them a fast answer or email them the proper ideas or systems to correct their issue and get the "yes" they were looking for. They were always grateful.

Now, it's time to take my consultation work to the next level and help *you*!

What You'll Learn from this Book

By following my method, you (as the hygienist) become an entrepreneur, or a *"hygiene-preneur,"* in your department, your practice, and . . . your career. And you win. Every time. This is the real deal.

So what will you learn? Here's what my method teaches:

1. You'll learn to establish a *hygiene mission statement*, and why it's vital.
2. You'll learn the steps and key components that produce positive outcomes.
3. You'll learn the importance of controlling new and existing patient experiences, and of getting the assessment right.
4. You'll master the skills for presenting a treatment plan so that you can always "get the yes."

5.   You'll learn to think beyond what you can do for your patients in order to reach a standard that's above "the usual."

6.   You'll learn to enhance your level of care by offering adjunct procedures that will improve your patients' health in addition to your own profitability per appointment.

7.   You'll learn how to schedule appropriately for what your patient needs and work more efficiently while generating more income per appointment.

8.   You'll learn how to become the manager of your own schedule so you can truly be a Hygienepreneur.

9.   And, finally, you'll learn to show how your special relationship with your patients can keep them active and "in your chair" for many years.

In addition, this guide will teach awesome "recall and reactivation" skills to decrease your rate of attrition and keep your schedule full, which will ultimately increase your personal income. The goal: two hygienists for every doctor. When you have this dynamic in place, the doctor's schedule is supported and the daily practice goals are met with ease. As a hygienist, you'll see big payoffs in return.

One great way of achieving the American Dream is by contributing something worthwhile to society, while at the same time making more money (while working less). If you're a hygienist, this book is the ultimate guide to helping make those dreams come true for you.

Now, let me tell you how the dream came true for me.

A Life-Changing Realization

A few years ago, my life was at a turning point. I was a single mom, busy supporting my children's dreams and goals. I was working in Southern California, where I had grown up. In my own eyes, I was living the dream—I was part of a successful dental practice, working for someone I considered the best doctor in the world. My children and I had beaten the odds. It all seemed like it was working out.

But not really. Everything I'd worked for was on the verge of crashing down around me.

With all the stress of my life, over the years I had unfortunately leaned on food as a crutch. I was really unhealthy, despite accomplishing many professional goals. The harsh reality? I weighed 289 pounds—about 160 pounds over the weight that I should have been. I was a ticking time bomb. Something had to change.

To understand how I got to that point, let me first say that I am the product of two very hard-working parents. My father was an executive chef who always worked three jobs to make ends meet, and my mother was in the catering and the food industries. My parents both worked fourteen-hour days without blinking an eye or complaining. I learned early that if I wanted anything in life I would have to work hard and be self-made.

Growing up, I was expected to figure out my life plan pretty quickly. My parents were tough: nothing was to be done with half of an effort. To be sure, I was loved and was taught good lessons early on, lessons that would stay ingrained in me forever. But we were never allowed to cut corners and there was very little praise given: high performance was simply expected.

After high school, my parents' career choices influenced me. I decided early on that I would go into the customer service industry at a restaurant or hotel/resort. And so I landed a great job at La Costa Resort and Spa in Carlsbad, CA. I worked everywhere on the La Costa property—on the golf course, in every restaurant, and I even catered to the needs of our successful private members. I loved it! Making the guests happy during their stays was an absolute pleasure. I found that I was quite good at it as well. As employees, we were "on stage" while serving our guests. We had to look a certain way. We presented ourselves for duty with a fresh face and always with an inviting smile. I was in the business of making others feel comfortable and happy.

I knew that catering to the needs of others fulfilled me and it made me feel good to serve. I excelled in this environment but wanted to move up in the resort industry world. The Ritz-Carlton was calling my name! When I had the opportunity to work for this wonderful company, I knew that I was on my way. So, at that time, I decided to go back to school to study hotel management. It meant being far away from my large family, but I knew there was much to gain by making the sacrifice.

All alone, I moved to Palm Springs, CA, and lived with no furniture in a vacant house that my Uncle owned, starting at the Ritz-Carlton as a concierge. I went through their extensive training program and learned how to raise the guest experience to a whole other level of customer care. The five-star touch was learned and practiced through my words and actions. They taught me communication skills that would later help me in every aspect of my life, both personal and professional.

The "Ritz-Carlton Way" was amazing. I was transformed as a person and I carried myself in a more confident way because of the skills they taught me. However, coming from a large family, I was terribly homesick in Palm Springs. I knew no one and the house was lonely without my family. I was happy professionally but miserable personally. Struggling with this, I decided to move back home to San Diego. And that's how I fell into the dentistry profession.

Beginning a Career in Dentistry

It all started after I moved back home, at a routine dental cleaning appointment with my family's new dentist. She was so nice and asked a lot of questions about my life as a young person and about my goals. After moving home, I also had met someone, fallen in love, and was ready to start a family. As a result of this newfound change, I'd decided to set aside my dreams of college and working in the resort service industry. During my next dental cleaning visit, I mentioned that I wanted to be married and have children. My dentist said that my communication skills were impressive and that I was bright, and she asked me if I had ever thought about dentistry as a career.

I hadn't, but she offered to train me if I went to work for her in her front office, part time. She said that the skills I had learned at high-end resorts like La Costa and the Ritz-Carlton could be transferred to the dental practice environment. I was intrigued and decided to accept the position she offered. I did not realize how fascinating this new field would be for me!

I put school on hold to learn everything I could about the front office part of the dental business. There was so much to know! I went to countless continuing education classes on dental billing, scheduling, insurance contract negotiations, and clinical dental topics. Like a sponge, I soaked up the lessons and loved it—I truly started to soar. I could not get enough dental knowledge. She allowed me to assist and see procedures up close. It was exciting! She would take a broken tooth and make it beautiful, fearful patients and calm them. I was able to use what I'd learned about communication at the Ritz-Carlton to help her with this, and soon I found I was helping to build her dental business.

I was able to collect money from patients with no issues—they even thanked me for doing so! I was able to calm down patients who were unhappy, whether it was about an insurance issue or some other problem. The dentist was able to focus on dentistry, and I handled the other aspects of her business. I grew from these experiences and, after a while, felt confident that it was time to move to a larger practice to see what I could accomplish on a bigger stage.

I moved on to work in practices that accepted HMO insurance as well as private insurance. Some of them had up to sixteen operatories, and one of the doctors owned three practices that also provided specialty care. I quickly moved into a position as a regional manager, where I ran six offices, handling all staffing, payroll, training, insurance contract negotiations, and the daily business operations.

It was rewarding and fast paced and I loved it! My "American Dream" was in sight. By that time I was married, had a young child, and was making a decent income without a college degree. I worked just like my parents did: twelve-to-fourteen hours a day, without complaining. The six dental offices were productive and I was running them like efficient machines—all at the age of twenty-five! The needs of the doctor, of my team, and of the patients were all being met and I was happy . . . for the time being. Then, all of a sudden, my marriage ended and I found myself the single parent of two small children.

It was a "fight or flight" situation. In order to not lose everything, I had to make smart decisions for myself and my children. Being self-sufficient and having a strong work ethic, I moved forward and maneuvered my way into another career change. I was divorced, with a three year old and a five year old, living in Temecula, CA and working fifty miles south, in San Diego. I had to change jobs in order to be closer to my children. So, I took a new job managing a dental office in Temecula and began training to become a hygienist.

Becoming a Dental Hygienist . . . and an Entrepreneur

I worked for a very encouraging dentist who allowed me to manage his successful private practice and tailor my hours around a busy, full-time school schedule. Having seen the various careers in a dental practice from within, I knew that next to being a dentist, a dental hygiene career was the next best thing in terms of compensation. Being a hygienist would also allow me to give my children the time that they deserved while helping me generate the income I needed to support them. So, the decision was made: I was "on fire"—ready to do whatever it took to meet this next challenge!

I took care of my kids, and also worked and went to school full time. My children were now seven and nine and showing advanced interest in athletics, playing baseball and softball year-round. But the truth was clear—our lives "were running us." It took me a long time to get through all of the prerequisites for dental hygiene school, but I finally got them all completed and applied for admission. My goal was to become a practicing dental hygienist as quickly as possible. After all, I had to work and provide for my children. My family was not in a position to help me financially.

My family did give me something more important, though—the gift of a work ethic and the will to fight for what I wanted. These life lessons empowered me to apply to a fast-track hygiene program that would allow me to finish in record time so I could start working. I wanted to complete hygiene school and become a great hygiene provider, and to help build dental practices. After all, I had already done that several times. I was good at it and confident that I could help my doctors become successful. Only this time, rather than doing it from the front of the practice, I'd be doing it from the back!

This was the Big Idea. Using my systematic approach with dental hygiene, I could build a department and then repeat this methodology over and over again. I could train other hygienists to follow the systems that I created and that were proven to work. This repeatable, trainable hygiene success program would enable a dentist to build his practice and, if he wanted to, easily sell it. I was going to be a new type of hygienist—a dynamic, super-powered dental hygienist. I knew the plan and I was on my way!

Luckily, I was quickly accepted into a program. It was very difficult, both financially and physically. I had to juggle my studies, my bills, and my children's school and sports schedules. But after sixteen months, and a few extra months waiting on multiple exam results, I did it—I was licensed to practice and was able to get to work and provide for my children.

Now I was officially a dental hygienist, but it felt much the same as when I became a mother—I had all the working parts but not much "know how." No one gave me the ultimate handbook on how to be great at either. I needed some time to grow personally and professionally. To see what type of practice I wanted to work in, I decided to take some temporary dental jobs in general practices, as well as specialties of pediatrics and periodontics. Through trial and error, I discovered my own way of practicing dental hygiene, and decided that the general practice environment would best fuel my goal for "practice building."

Bottom line: It took many twists and turns to become the hygiene provider that I am today. My success seems easy now because I practice the same way every day, and I always win. I've successfully taken the front office management tools that I used for over twenty years and merged them into the practice of dental hygiene, and it has truly been a winning combination. I became the Hygienepreneur that I always wanted to be!

But I still had to get healthy.

Taking Care of Myself—for a Change

I had accomplished a lot, but it would all be for nothing if I didn't do something about my weight. I suffered from hypertension, and I was on medications like hydrochlorothiazide and lisinopril. The reality check came when we were testing patients with a prescreening for sleep apnea and I decided to test myself, to serve as a good example.

The readings were terrible: I had a bad case. It forced my dentist to refer me to a pulmonologist in town for further testing. The pulmonologist read my initial screening results and gave me equipment to use to do further testing during a night of sleep. It showed that I did indeed have sleep apnea and, at the age of just forty-two, he wanted me to wear a *continuous positive airway pressure* (CPAP) therapy machine every night. My weight was so high and my health was so bad, I realized, I would have to wear a machine to simply breathe at night, maybe for the rest of my life. With sleep apnea, I would literally stop breathing at night repeatedly while I was sleeping.

It shocked me. I had gained weight and lost weight like crazy over the years, but this was my rock bottom. I'd tried everything from Nutrisystem to Weight Watchers and doctor-managed programs, but they all left me feeling upset and defeated, even though normally I was a very positive person. It wasn't that I was lazy, but I lacked discipline and was focused on the others around me, like my family and my practice, rather than my own needs. I had to face the facts: this problem I had with food was bigger than I could handle. Nothing was working.

I did not have much money—nor did I come from money. But my little family had reached its goals, right? My education and career were on track, both of my children got the college athletic scholarships they wanted. I was still living in my home, which I fought tooth and nail to keep. However, this silent killer was breathing down my neck. The truth:

I was on track to miss out on the fruits of my labor, because I would not be alive to enjoy it.

The answer? Surgery. It seemed like the only thing that would deliver the results that I so desperately needed.

Weight loss surgery had never been an option for me before. I had struggled to lose weight for years. My cousin had undergone the surgery and had been successful with it, but I never thought it was how I would ultimately get the weight off. I had never had any kind of surgery before, but something had to be done. I started by asking my favorite nurse practitioner about the pros and cons of having the surgery. She looked into my health history and my current condition and guided me through the rigorous process of getting the surgery approved by my insurance company.

There were definite guidelines to follow to get the authorizations in order. First, I had to participate in a medically supervised weight loss program for six months, with documentation of doctor appointments completed along the way. I had to show proof that I had tried alternative measures to lose the weight. Second, I suffered from two or more comorbidities and had to be on multiple medications. I had to see a psychiatrist who could evaluate whether or not I would have post-surgery success and could handle the mental struggle of it all and not gain the weight back. I also had to attend seminars, workshops, and classes on the different surgical options that were available to me on the management of my body and life after the surgery. I sent blood samples to labs as well as procedures and tests such as an electrocardiogram, chest X ray, CT scans, and MRIs. They showed I had an extremely fatty liver and that it was quite possible that I would need my gallbladder removed. I was a mess.

It took so much time to get through the requirements to satisfy the insurance company that I almost lost hope after ten months of waiting. Then I got a phone call that would change my life.

The weight-loss doctor (my hero!) called my work phone number to tell me that the surgery was finally approved and they had a surgery date in mind. I know it sounds crazy, but by then it had been so long since I'd first started the process that I began having doubts about doing it at all. I had lost twelve pounds from the six-month weight loss program. For a minute, I thought I might just keep doing that. I was, of course, trying to back out of it. After I hung up the phone, I even told my front office scheduler that I was having doubts—they wanted to do it in November (and it was October), and we were just too busy at work with the holidays coming up. I didn't want to inconvenience the practice by being off at our busiest time of the year, or recuperating during the holidays. Maybe I would just do it next year, I thought.

That was silly, she said. They would manage all right without me. I should just get it done. I said I better ask the doctor's permission because I was his biggest producer and I was always concerned about the loss of business when I took time off. He was in the office lab, so I went back there to talk to him.

He was working on a denture at the time. "Can we talk? I asked. I proceeded to tell him that I'd been approved, but the surgery date they were proposing would be in November. "Okay," he said. "Great! Make sure to tell the scheduling coordinator and we will get it all worked out." With tears rushing down my face, I told him that I understood if he wanted to recommend a better date. "No," he said. "You need to do this, Tiffany. You will do just fine, and our office will be okay while you are gone. It is time for you to take care of yourself."

So I did it.

A New Life, a New Me

I was super nervous—the weight-loss doctor told me I had to lose weight before the surgery or he would cancel it. Apparently my liver was so big that I had to shrink it so that he could operate around my vital organs without fear of complications. I had already lost twelve pounds but had to lose almost thirty in order to be ready. When the day finally arrived, my mother took me to the medical facility—the Bariatric Center for Excellence at Parkview Community Hospital Medical Center, in Riverside, CA. I checked in, weighed in, and lo and behold I had accomplished the goal! I'd lost the full thirty pounds, so the nurse said she could finish checking me in and prepare me for surgery. I was scared but excited when they wheeled me in.

I woke up in the weight-loss surgery wing of the clinic, tired and in lots of pain. My first thought was the same one I'd had when I quit my job and found myself sitting in a classroom on the first day of dental hygiene school: *What have I done?* Maybe I had messed up my life! Then I saw my mother's sweet face, and I shared my worries with her. "No, honey," she said. "You have done the right thing. You have taken the first step to truly changing your life and living longer."

She was right: I had to live a long life for my children, and I didn't want to die young. I was going to beat this weight loss challenge—it was like a fire inside me! My two children were collegiate athletes by now, very fit and strong individuals, and their example drove me. I'd hired personal trainers for both of them as they progressed in their sports, and now it was my turn. I hired my daughter's athletic trainer, the same one who prepared her for college softball, and I did amazingly well with his guidance.

I worked out four to five days a week and wrote down every ounce of liquid or food that entered my body. I took my special supplements and kept in close contact with my weight loss support nurse. I lost one to one-and-a-half pounds every day. Eventually, the weight was practically falling off of me. I purchased cheap clothes from Walmart because they would only fit for a couple of weeks before I would have to wear a different size. It was invigorating to donate the clothes that did not fit me anymore to charity. In the beginning, I was a size twenty-six. Never again! I even went down a shoe size.

Looking back now, I truly appreciate the medical team that helped me lose 158 pounds in the year after I made the decision to have surgery. That decision did not come easy. As a single person who was the primary earner for her children, I was concerned about the loss of work time, the loss of income, and—most concerning—whether I would die during surgery, leaving my children without their mother. But I made it, and I'm better than ever now. God is good.

Flash forward to the present day, and I am now a size six and feel great! The weight loss surgery was on November 20, 2015. It has been almost six years since I had the surgery and when people ask me if I would do it again I always say yes. I am not looking back. My life has changed dramatically for the better, forever.

The challenges that I had as a heavier person no longer define me: I can ride on an airplane and sit in the seat comfortably. My food bill has decreased; because I had gastric bypass surgery, I can only eat a small amount of food at a time, so I never eat sweets, fried foods, or drink carbonated drinks, and I'm very selective about which restaurants I choose to eat at. It's easier to shop, too—especially for clothes. I have more options and they're more affordable!

My life is wonderful! I have no health limitations to inhibit me from the next phase in my career, the phase that I am being called for. What is that exactly?

You're reading it.

The Mission of a Hygienepreneur

Life sometimes seems like it's all timing, doesn't it? Now that my children are grown and are done playing college baseball and softball, and both have their degrees, it is *my time*.

I very much want to empower others who need a lift in life. I want to share the challenges I have faced to help other dental hygienists in their life journeys. This is my calling, and is the next step in what I need to do to give back to this industry that has given so much to me.

As a strong, traditionally raised woman who believes in the foundation of family, I believe in a family dynamic where the husband and wife support and respect one another. Fortunately, I witnessed this in practice growing up, which was a beautiful thing to see. When life circumstances forced me to be a single mother for over twenty years, I had to dig deep, be strong, and make sacrifices to raise my children in a nurturing and winning environment. In life, sometimes women are forced to do more on their own than they expected growing up. Not only can divorce happen, but spouses can get sick—even pass away. When a woman is left destitute by a devastating change in life, whatever her struggle may be, I want to do whatever I can to help.

One thing I can do is help hygienists become *Hygienepreneurs like me*!

My mission now is to embrace hygienists—especially women—who have encountered imperfect life circumstances and support them and guide them into a world of success and confidence and independence for themselves and for those they love. By encouraging them, and teaching the practices that made me a Hygienepreneur, I can help my fellow sister (and brother) hygienists rise above any and all circumstances, find happiness, and ultimately, win. When done right, the Hygienepreneur's tactical approach operates like a smooth-running machine that enhances your doctor's success, and consequently yours as well. To be "hygiene driven" is the key for dental practices. When it pays off (and it will) your doctor can relax a little and let a strong, powerful team of hygienists lead the way.

So, developing other Hygienepreneurs is what is next for me. After I share "the way" I developed, you and your doctor will come to appreciate how a hygienist's systematic approach can lead to increased patient care and increased production. With my proven methodology, everyone truly wins.

It's a fact: doctors absolutely need to use their hygienists to drive their practices' growth. A long time ago, I discovered that adopting and executing certain systems will ensure both provider and patient with "a win" every time. This book helps put that idea into practice. Each of the chapters in the book is filled with useful, practical information that can positively drive your practice to great heights. Knowing your numbers and where you stand hourly, daily, and monthly is half the battle. After that, it's all gravy—meaning goals have been met and all that is extra should be yours to celebrate.

Now, let's get to work.

I. SETTING THE FOUNDATION

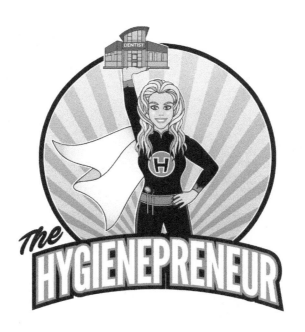

CHAPTER 1
The Dental Hygiene Mission Statement: Making the Vision a Reality

The start of your "pyramid of success" is, of course, the foundation. That foundation is a mission statement—not the mission statement of the whole dental practice, but the hygiene department's mission statement. What are the beliefs of our department? Why do we exist and what are our purposes and goals for our patients? The statement should answer those questions.

Decide your principles in advance, as a team. Working with the doctor, the hygienists should decide together what the overall goals should be for their patients, and set up the standard of care protocols to meet those goals. After you've established the mission statement, then comes the assessment, periodontal classification, and the method of care for each patient. If you decide on these criteria in advance and they are established as the foundation of the hygiene appointment, then all providers will be in sync and will be calibrated when delivering the proper care to each patient.

By establishing a mission statement you will establish a direction that will enhance patient care, streamline work performance and increase profitability. You'll see a reduction of stress, and an increase in time spent with patients. Whether you have veteran hygienists in your practice or newbies, the blended consensus should be unified. All clinicians in the practice should take the same path as far as patient care is concerned and follow the same assessment patterns and care plans customized for the specific condition.

Elements of a Mission Statement

Your mission statement should include a mission defined by values and vision (Fig. 1.1).

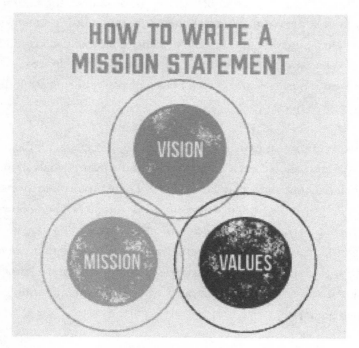

Fig. 1.1 — Writing a mission statement

In regards to the dental hygiene mission statement, my doctor, K. Pat

Brown, DDS told me that "the first step in a hygiene-driven practice is to realize that hygiene is so important to the practice it needs its own mission and vision statements."

The doctor and the hygienists can create the mission statement (or *hygiene credo*) together. You'll want to decide these things in advance:

- How to categorize your patients
- What recommendations to give for treating the periodontal needs of patients in each periodontal classification.
- What recall (cleaning schedule) each classification type should be put on
- What adjuncts and hygiene aids should be encouraged for each patient

But first, what is your mission statement? What is the standard of care for hygiene that you want to target and live by? The dental hygiene credo is the foundation for "everything hygiene" in your practice. So let's write it!

The Dental Hygiene Credo

Here's an example of a mission statement, or hygiene credo, from my practice:

Mission   *To provide each patient with the perfect, over the top, 5-star, red carpet experience.*

The K. Pat Brown DDS Dental Hygiene Team strives to maintain a place where the genuine care and comfort of our patients is our highest priority. Whole health and advanced hygiene practices are utilized to combat disease. We shall serve our patients in the fullest capacity using a non-lecturing and gentle approach to communication.

Vision   ***Utilizing top technology, skill, and in partnership with our patients, we will maintain and protect the oral foundation to protect against the destruction of gum and bone. We strive to manage and maintain pocket probing depths to eliminate 100 percent of all gingival inflammation to protect our patients' overall body wellness.***

We will gently educate all new patients and existing patients about the highest standards of care and share our core values of being proactive in dental health to promote overall body health.

Values   ***We commit to serve our patients with the utmost respect and will strive to listen to our patients' wishes and concerns and values. We will be united in our philosophy of our message and in our treatment recommendations.***

Purpose of the Mission and Vision Statements

Mark A. Costes, DDS, a well-known dentist and author of *Pillars of Dental Success*, puts it this way:

While the purpose of the Mission Statement is to clearly define why a company exists, a Vision Statement addresses where your company is going. The vision statement serves as the inspiration for what you and the team strive to accomplish on a daily basis and guides your long-term strategic planning.

The mission statement for your hygiene department will aid in establishing the direction of care for your patients. What does the team want to accomplish? What are your goals for your patients and what are the hygiene outcomes that you want to strive for? When you answer these questions, then your mission statement will be complete. The end goal? Your mission statement will be the foundation that you can build upon, the philosophy that drives your practice. After all, just about every major company has a mission statement as its foundation (Fig. 1.2).

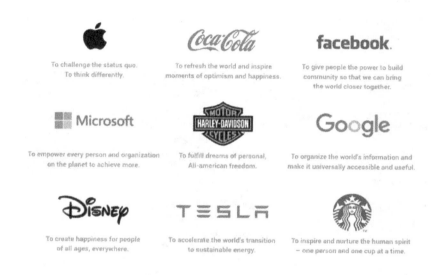

Figure 1.2 — Mission statements for major brands

Benefits of a Mission Statement

Create a mission statement and you will see your level of patient care become truly awesome! Your patients want this from you. Always give them the best of everything that is offered in your practice and you will gain their loyalty and trust. As hygienists, we must all be united with the need for a hygiene credo.

In addition, unity in the practice will reduce confusion between team members and will give the patient security knowing that the dental team that he has entrusted his dental care with is taking care of him in every possible way. When we operate with confidence, the patient will have confidence and trust in us. It's all about our culture. Big or small, customer-service-based businesses that are successful (Fig. 1.3) all include the same ingredient: a solid culture. Create this in your environment and you will win.

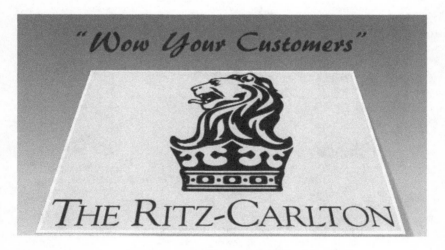

Figure 1.3 — The Ritz-Carlton Way

Creating an exceptional culture that builds a cohesive organization may take time and a long-term commitment, but the payoff to any brand or company is felt through the customer experience.
—The Ritz-Carlton Way

CHAPTER 2
Assessing the New and Existing Patient

Once you have your mission statement completed, one of your most important tools (Fig. 2.1) will be your hygiene care protocol. It should help you decide what it will all mean when you assess a patient and develop the care plan. After you've laid the foundation of the mission statement, the hygiene care protocol builds on it with an assessment for new and existing patients. Everything rests on getting the patient assessed and cared for correctly.

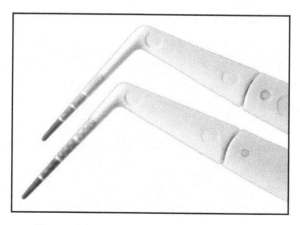

Figure 2.1 — Dental periodontal probe

How will you do it? You'll need to decide your approach methodically and then go for it!

In baseball, the pitcher and the catcher need to be in sync. If they are not fluid and on the same page, the team will lose the game. The same holds true for the dentist and hygienist. Whether it's a new patient or an existing patient who needs a re-assessment, the key to success is continuity and calibration. The dentist and hygienists all need to be on the same page.

Different Approaches to Assessments

I have worked for many dental practices with different dentists who have different approaches regarding restorative care and hygiene care. Not every doctor practices the same way or has the same beliefs about when to treat an area and when not to. I am sure you have experienced different doctor philosophies of when to observe an area of the mouth or treat it. Some doctors will be more proactive on an incipient area of decay, where others will simply monitor it. It is all in their approach and what they are feeling at the time.

As hygienists, we are there to support doctors' findings and their plans for the patient. But if we are not on the same page as our doctor, then where does that leave the patient? As hygienists, we will get more case acceptance if we concur with our doctor.

So, doctors, how do you accomplish a unified approach in your practice? It clearly takes time. And it takes a lot of discussion: you have to put in the work together for a few months. Whether it is the multi-doctor practice team sitting down with its hygienists and going through a few cases, or a single-doctor practice using a case by case approach with each hygienist, this exercise needs to be completed. The doctors should be calibrated as far as their approach and care, and the hygienists need to know at all times what the doctor is going to recommend as a treatment plan for a patient.

Getting the assessment right for new and existing patients, according to K. Pat Brown, DDS, is necessary because "your approach to periodontal health will change throughout your career, as will the treatments available. Therefore, we should not diagnose once and treat based on the same treatment forever. Create clear protocols and reevaluate them once a year with your hygiene team."

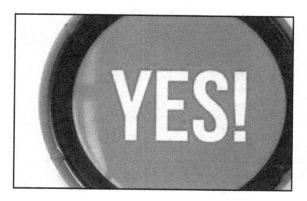

Figure 2.2 — Getting the "yes"

Anticipating our doctor's needs is key. We can anticipate and prepare more thoroughly if we already know what our doctors are going to suggest. We need to prepare to practice with ease. We need to practice like an athlete getting ready for the big game—the big event is the patient visit, and we need to bring our "A" game to the field to get the home run and score the "yes" from our patient (Fig. 2.2). Setting aside time to go through a few cases together will ensure that everybody is on board and knows the approach the doctor will take.

Show and Tell

As the hygienist, whether for an existing patient or new patient, you need to tell them the areas that you see as potential concerns. Let them know that you are seeing an issue with a tooth, or an area, and indicate that the doctor will be looking at it as well. The intraoral camera (Fig. 2.3) should be utilized to take pictures of these areas of concern before the doctor comes in to complete the diagnosis.

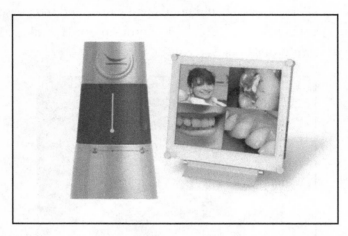

Figure 2.3 — Intraoral camera

Gary Kadi, Author of *Million Dollar Dentistry*, offers this advice:

Dust off your intraoral camera and ensure your hygienist has at least four shots of problem areas up when the doctor enters the hygiene room for a re-care visit. Chances are that you already have an intraoral camera, which offers a ten-times-actual-size blowup of situations in a patient's mouth. Big, flat-screen TVs are very inexpensive, and on them decay looks like the Grand Canyon, and as for gum recession . . . there aren't any words. Most dentists have intraoral cameras, yet few of them use these expensive devices. If you don't show the patient what's unhealthy, how could the patient possibly understand the nature of the problem? That's actually the job of the hygienist, so that by the time the dentist comes into the room, all the dentist has to do is go over the necessary treatment instead of wasting valuable time convincing the patient that there really is a problem.

Put these pictures in front of patients for them to see. Let them know that this is a potential problem area and communicate that you will assess whether it needs care at this time or not. When the doctor comes into your room, let them know what you have seen and what you and the patient have discussed. Tell the doctor that you have already shown your patient the photos and ask him his opinion. Take X rays as well, if need be. This is a great setup for your doctor to be able to come in and easily "knock it out of the park." Your goal is to make his job easier.

Since you are finding potential issues and sharing the information, your doctor will become more confident in your ability. The patient's needs are well taken care of because you both are operating like a "well-oiled" machine. You are very important in this scenario and need to showcase your exceptional skills. Then the doctor can decide what he wants to treat and what he doesn't want to treat. The fact that you have brought patient issues to his attention up front is a plus for everyone.

At my practice, our patients love our suggestions because they love us. A good hygienist is valued by their patients. Consider this: have you ever had a patient ask you if they truly need to complete the care that was recommended after the doctor completes the exam? It happens to me all of the time. In most cases, a hygienist's word is "gold" to the patient's ears.

Calibration and Unity

This all starts with calibration and unity. It benefits the patient if you and your doctor are in agreement, because, after all, four eyes are better than two eyes, right? The skill that that we, as hygienists, have is awesome. Because of our extensive schooling and experience in the field, we can pre-assess a patient very accurately. We should always be very thorough in our approach; when we are, this will help the doctor tremendously. So as a hygienist, make sure that you are on the same page with your doctor and the way he approaches his care. Along with calibrating with the doctor, the hygiene team needs to be calibrated as a unit, but it all starts with calibration between the dentist and the hygienist.

Just as the hygienist should tune in to the doctor's preferred method on how to approach the patient's restorative needs, the hygienist and doctor need to share the same method when it comes to the patient's hygiene care. This approach needs to be looked at in advance, and through multiple case evaluations. Going through cases in advance together as a team, sharing the assessment process and the approach that should be taken for that patient, is of great value to the practice. If the entire practice is on the same page, uses the same approach, and knows how to take care of each patient effectively, then the patient wins. Knowing eliminates guessing.

A planned hygiene system at your practice, when followed by all, reduces confusion and stress in the office. As clinicians, we operate more productively and systematically when everyone is practicing the same. So, the calibration between doctor and hygienist is key, but the calibration between hygienists in the office is extremely important as well.

Developing Hygiene Protocols

So how do you do that? First, develop the hygiene system and protocols that the office is going to follow. Put together a flowchart on one sheet that shows a patient assessment, the different periodontal categories (Fig. 2.4), and the care plan that should be followed for each category. This care plan should include any adjuncts, plus the recommended recall for your patients.

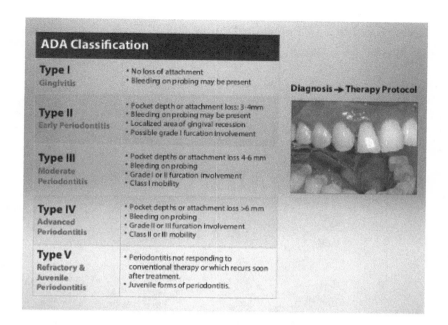

Figure 2.4 —
American Dental Association Periodontal Classifications

Whatever the system is, make sure that it is right for your office and is followed the same way by each provider. Look, we were all taught in school how to assess the patient properly. The key is to stop doing the "bloody prophy." Doing a standard cleaning on a patient who has periodontal probing depths that are indicative of disease (plus bone loss) is an accident waiting to happen. We need to make it clear that this type of substandard care will not be practiced on our watch. We now know that oral inflammation can be associated with inflammation in other parts of the body. Preventing other health issues like diabetes, heart problems and occurrence of strokes is how we can do our part to save lives.

In their excellent book, *Hygiene Superstar* (Fig. 2.5), Mike Czubiak, DDS and Steve Sperry write, "[Researchers] know that so much death and disability are caused by inflammation and as it turns out, the mouth is a huge source of that inflammation. Hundreds of studies have shown that periodontal disease is a root cause of systemic inflammation."

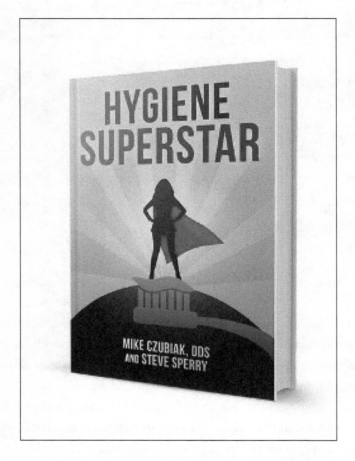

Figure 2.5 — Mike Czubiak, DDS and Steve Sperry's book, *Hygiene Superstar*

Delivering the Message

We need to not be afraid to deliver the message about periodontal disease and the need for extra care. If we are all following the same direction in the appropriate lane there will be no accidents. The system should be followed the same way every time, by every provider. However, we have all been faced with that hygiene provider who is resistant to change and does not think that the care direction that the rest of the team developed is one that she or he should follow. Such a hygienist resists new technologies and tools shared for treating gum infection. I often hear from doctors who are struggling with a hygienist who resists offering adjuncts and services that may not be covered by a patient's insurance. They ask, "how do I get my hygienist on board like the others? She always says that she is not comfortable 'selling' dentistry."

Here is a clue: The way to present the change to this provider is not by discussing the financial benefits to the practice at first. We should present the changes for what they are: a specific procedure that will benefit that patient's oral health. If we present the systemic benefits of adding a procedure to an appointment, the hygienist will get on board like the others. Be sure to stress the clinical benefits. Highlight the fact that you are now in the business of overall systemic health, not just oral health. Then, to support this hygienist and get her total commitment for other patients moving forward, send her to classes on overall systemic health that starts with oral health. She will be more open to the change, which helps everyone's well-being. Once all of your providers are "ready to rock" the new hygiene culture, you can streamline and unify the assessment system. The goal: a unified hygiene team and unified language used to deliver recommended care to the patient.

Our language should also be customized to the doctor's personal philosophy, and the same language needs to be adopted in the delivery of the message by every provider. A hygienist should complete the assessment and recommend a treatment plan to the doctor, and doctors should verify and approve the plan and support the hygienist with affirming words in front of the patient. If you are both saying the same thing, the patient feels secure and will be more willing to say "yes" to whatever plan you are recommending. Start with the assessment, then gather the data to support the findings.

Documenting Protocols

The assessment process has a lot of inputs and variables that make it truly amazing when it all comes together and is completed for a patient. Remember, don't forget to have a team meeting internally to decide on the system and protocol that your office wants to follow. This system needs to be preset, and the parameters documented accordingly with a flowchart-style diagram.

For example:

- IF the patient has a certain amount of bloody 5+mm pocket charting with x amount of bone loss,
- THEN the patient will be placed in a certain category of perio types,
- AND scaling and root planing will be completed,
- AND a three-month recall schedule will be recommended.

With this specific care plan, laser disinfection and/or antibiotic therapy may be necessary as well.

Mike Czubiak, DDS and Steve Sperry write,

> During scaling and root planing or a maintenance visit, we must focus on reducing pathogenic bacteria. Of course, deplaquing and deposit removal is still important, but the goal has totally changed. And success is not measured by lack of bone loss, but by eradicating inflammation. You've probably had one of those patients with bright red, puffy bleeding gums but not a lot of deposits. What's going on? Inflammation! And going only after the deposits and telling the patient to floss more just isn't enough. It just doesn't work. I think we have all been there.

Also, adult fluoride varnish treatments can be added to reduce sensitivity and aid in the prevention of decay and remineralization. The recommended tools and home care products can also be established as the standard recommendations of the practice as well.

For example, if the patient is classified as a periodontally involved patient, then the practice will uniformly recommend a WaterPik and electric toothbrush, or interproximal go-between brushes and an electric toothbrush and floss. The team can decide in advance and establish which care plan they want to follow per patient type. The point is to establish your perio parameters in advance and follow the plan to its entirety throughout the practice. In a multi-provider practice, this is crucial. However, by pre-setting the guidelines and the care that corresponds with them, the patients' needs are met and their periodontal health stays managed. The patient is now under a complete comprehensive care plan that will ensure success that everyone will be pleased to see. Remember, too, that patient records are always best presented when the images are updated and complete.

The images for a patient include both intraoral pictures and traditional radiographs. These pictures for new and existing patients should always be updated so that the patient continues to be assessed correctly. The X rays are not just used for detection of caries, but can be utilized to compare whether bone levels are changing or staying the same over time. Before patients arrive, the front office should verify the patients' insurance benefits and X-ray histories. You should always take whatever X rays are necessary with the patient's permission, whether they are covered by insurance or not, but it is easier when we are able to predetermine insurance coverage so we can inform the patient. At the office I currently work at, if the full-mouth X rays are needed but were previously done at another office, and can't be quickly obtained, we frequently do them as a courtesy in order to complete comprehensive treatment plans. This should be a predetermined practice protocol. X rays are necessary to ensure a complete diagnosis and increase patient care.

The frequency of patients' X rays should be established as well. Every patient should be placed on an individualized X ray schedule. A patient who has low caries and little-to-no bone loss should have less frequent X rays than a patient who has bone loss and a high frequency of caries. This guideline can be discussed and monitored by the doctor. The key is to agree in advance what the hygiene program is for your office and have every provider follow it to its entirety. It's key to utilize your imaging system to solidify what you already see with the patient.

X rays and current intraoral images are very important when evaluating such things as bone health and calculus buildup. Intraoral images are ideal for showing the patient and the insurance company the need for the appropriate care. Also, it is very revealing to compare the first images taken to those that are taken one, three, and ten years later, and to see that the bone level has not changed and that the care plan that you and the patient are following is working.

Building Patient Understanding

Show the patients their X rays and show them their bone level. If patients understand a little bit about what they are seeing, it will back up what you are recommending to them. They need to be told that X rays are not just for diagnosing decay and oral needs, but that they are an important part of making sure that the bone is staying healthy and not changing. If a new patient comes into your practice and you show him or her bone levels that reveal early or moderate bone loss, it is important to say that you can keep it at that level for a long time with their help. Your patients won't be able to get that bone back, but reassure them that you can help them to not lose more—if they follow your recommended care.

Explain to them that your goal is for their bone level to stay the same, and that if both of you follow the plan in the office and at home, then they will see success. Stress that you and the patient are a team, working in conjunction to make sure that that happens. This same point holds true for the healthy patient wanting to avoid the loss of tissue attachment. Encourage them to use their tools at home and follow the recall schedule recommended to them by the doctor and hygienist. Remember, current X rays are necessary to ensure periodontal health.

If patients have personal reasons for refusing X rays, it is perfectly fine to ask what their reservations might be. If it is due to financial reasons and they do not have insurance, then you should still take the X rays as a courtesy to them. It is more important to provide the proper care and get the assessment right, and get the "yes" from them, than to get the fee for the X rays. Plus, telling patients not to worry about the fee, and that you will do the X rays as a courtesy for them, will help build trust with those patients. This is a small way to build your practice from within. The patients will love you for it! But you should also educate them on the necessity of follow-up X rays, and the value of paying the fee.

If patients have other reservations or concerns, such as the safety of X rays, try to gently educate them on the need to optimize their health. Some patients say that they are concerned about radiation. If you use a digital X-ray system at the office, you can reassure your patient that the system's film speed is very fast and is quite safe, administering very low levels of radiation. Let patients know that the dentist can only see part of the tooth with the naked eye to formulate a diagnosis. Express this to patients, but work with them on establishing an X-ray completion schedule that will be satisfying to them without compromising their care.

If they refuse, you can say "yes" to not taking the X rays, but request that they get them done at their next recall to give you peace of mind in your diagnosis. It is okay to compromise with your patient and ask if the images can be done in three months. A patient is usually fine with this scenario. Plus, it makes patients feel that they are in charge and you are there to assist them with their care. Letting patients know that you are willing to work with them, but do not want to compromise their care, is important. We want to operate above the standard of care for their future health and are willing to do anything for them in order to meet and exceed these goals.

Intraoral images are an awesome way to show the patient their possible dental needs. The camera will show cracks in teeth, broken fillings, wear facets, and magnify cosmetic imperfections so that the patient can see them with the naked eye. An intraoral camera can also show the patient red bleeding gums, plaque levels, and tartar buildup that maybe they were not aware of. These pictures can be saved for future use. After their dental needs are met, new images can be taken to show a "before and after" scenario. After scaling and root planing, teeth should have no tartar and appear whiter. When before and after photos are placed side by side, it shows a great transformation. Also, a "before and after" X ray can help your patient see and confirm that your work was a job well done.

When tartar is present below the gum line, and then scaling and root planing is completed, the patient will be able to see that the tartar is gone and there is no more tartar on the tooth. This adds value to the care, and the patient will most likely develop a desire to not let it happen again. It also is a great tool to build trust between the practice and the patient. When patients can see what is wrong with a tooth and what the doctor's recommendations are for care, they are now involved in the decision making process for treating the area. They will be able to see what you are talking about and feel good about the care they are receiving.

Now, on to the assessment to get "the yes."

CHAPTER 3
Presenting Assessments with the Right Phrasing to "Get the Yes"

The final phase of the periodontal assessment, periodontal probing, should be spoken out loud for the patient to hear.

First, the hygienist should let the patient know that the gum exam assesses gum inflammation and loss of gum tissue—in plain language, you are checking for infection and disease. It is all part of making sure that there is adequate support for the teeth.

I have always told my patients that I like the numbers low: 2s and 3s are healthy numbers, while 4s mean gingivitis. Numbers that are 5 and above, we will talk about. I say these numbers out loud, and even say what areas are bleeding, while inputting them into the computer. Document and photograph recession areas and furcation involvements. If you find any teeth that are mobile, communicate that to the patient and record it. If exudate is present in the mouth, use the word "puss" with the patient.

Gathering all the information in the beginning helps the patient know which direction their care is going in. After the findings are complete, sit the patient up in the dental chair to deliver the message. This should be easy because they have been told what is happening and they've listened as you recorded their results. We also can show them the evidence of bone loss on the X ray, which is an awesome tool for validation. Intraoral images showing red gums and tartar can also inform the patient of what is present, conveying cause and effect. They already know the areas of concern.

Then explain to them that they are in good hands, and that based upon the numbers and what you are seeing, they are probably in need of more care than just a routine cleaning or prophy. Also, explain that if they have comorbidities like diabetes or other diseases, their need for care increases tremendously.

Mike Czubiak, DDS and Steve Sperry offer the following facts:

FACT: Treatment for periodontal disease is associated with a significantly reduced overall risk of cancer.

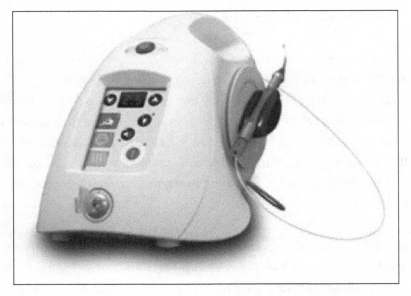

Figure 3.1 — Dental Laser Diode Soft Tissue Perio Surgical Kit

FACT: Treatment for periodontal disease leads to improved glycemic control in type 2 diabetic patients for at least three months.

FACT: Intensive periodontal treatment reduces systemic inflammatory markers and systolic blood pressure and improves lipid profiles.

Treatment planning for your patient is easy if you remember to do for them as if they were a family member. If they need a routine cleaning and they have 2s and 3s present, complete the cleaning and schedule them back for a six-month scheduled hygiene appointment. If they have evidence of bone loss and bleeding, 5s and 6s or more, then you know to bring them back or start that same day with limited or full-quadrant scaling and root planing.

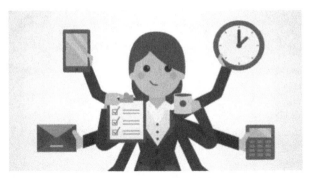

Figure: 3.2 — Scheduling

Laser disinfection (Fig. 3.1) or antibiotic therapy can be added to their treatment plan to improve periodontal health. Scheduling a patient back for this, as well as a six-week post-operation re-evaluation and three-month recall, is also a good idea and promotes retention. So add it from the beginning and explain it one time. You know it needs to be done, so tell them and save on words and time delivering the message. Get the "yes" in advance. This reduces your efforts during future visits (Fig. 3.2), all while increasing their periodontal health.

Pre booking hygiene appointments is a huge practice builder. No patient should ever leave without a reserved appointment. It is important to take the time yourself to schedule all of the hygiene appointments necessary to promote periodontal health, and also to fill your schedule! Only you know how much time you need to take care of all of the work for each of your patients. Being a Hygienepreneur requires you, as the hygienist, to be in charge of your schedule (Fig. 3.3).

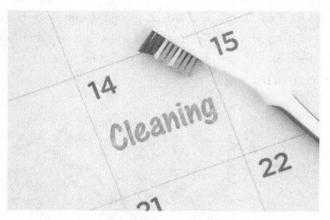

Figure 3.3 — Reserve it in advance

Along with planning the appropriate hygiene care for your specific case type, it is also important to pick and choose the appropriate hygiene-related adjunct procedures to enhance patients' health and the care you give them. You just need to say it to them and get "the yes." Seat patients upright in the dental chair (so they're eye to eye, knee to knee, heart to heart with you) to reassure them that this plan, which both you and the doctor have recommended, will ensure total perio-stability. This is a powerful moment between you and your patient. Always seize the opportunity!

Here is a script from a real-life scenario that happened recently between a patient and me:

HYGIENIST: "So, Mrs. Jones, we will of course confirm this with the doctor, but based on the teeth images, bone loss and tartar levels that we saw together today, we definitely need to see you back for special visits to combat the active disease. If it's okay with you, we are going to do a procedure called scaling and root planing. We will want to perform this procedure over two visits. We will numb your mouth for the procedure to ensure that you are comfortable. We will follow up the procedure with a laser to disinfect and reduce bacteria in the pockets and reduce inflammation and promote tightening of the tissue around the teeth.

After the procedure is done, we will follow up with a six-week checkup of the gums and place fluoride on all your teeth and root surfaces. This helps reduce the occurrence of sensitivity and recurrent decay. Afterwards, in order to maintain your perio health, we need to see you every three months to maintain your periodontal health.

A shorter cleaning schedule will help keep bacteria colonies under control and, in turn, will keep your bone levels stable. Preventing further destruction of bone and gum is key to ensuring that we will do everything in our power to prevent surgical solutions in the near future."

A Note on Scripting

In order to promote continuity and show that you are an expert, scripting is a valuable tool that is common in many businesses. I'll be talking about scripting throughout this book, and offering some tried and true scripts. We don't want to sound like robots, but having a guided script that we add our own flair to is crucial when promoting the yes!

If you practice scripting, your team will all be on the same page, and your patients will be more of a partner in their care plan because they will understand and accept the goals.

See *Appendix 1* for some helpful scripts.

The above example is how you should word it and communicate to your patients. It takes practice, but being specific with them and ensuring they understand will go a long way. They will be patients for life. When you start to see your team's mission statement and vision come to life, it is truly exciting. The team is calibrated with your doctor's visions for his patients and his hygiene practice is in motion. You are all on the same page and the patients' all feel confident under your care. Next, it is time to practice the techniques that keep your chairs filled with patients who trust and love you. Manage this and win again!

Now, on to **Part II**: Getting patients in the chair.

II. GETTING PATIENTS IN THE CHAIR

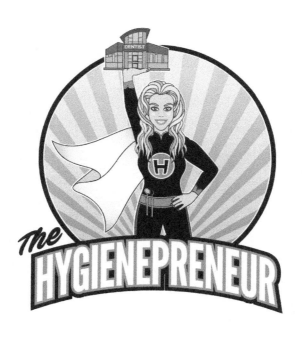

CHAPTER 4
The Patient Didn't Abandon You–Recall and Reactivation Tips

Managing recall can be easy when your daily hygiene reappointment rate is at 100%. Every hygienist should strive for that. In order to make sure that your schedule stays full, it is very important that every patient leaves with an appointment reserved for 3, 4 or 6 months out. If the patient is saying that they do not know their schedule in the future, reassure them that they can go ahead and schedule the appointment and change it if necessary when the date gets closer.

Since we all have access to the internet, no stone should be left unturned to gather information for that patient so that they are scheduled and locked in. If your patient is a college student who does not know his spring break schedule, take the time to look up the school calendar and schedule time when he is on break and will be home.

Pre-appointing the next hygiene appointment as part of a recall system is necessary so that your patients do not "fall through the cracks." Scheduling the appointment while they're still in your office is much easier than trying to chase them down later. Keeping your practice's attrition rate very low in order to help it grow is important (Fig. 4.1), and it is the hygienist's responsibility to make that happen.

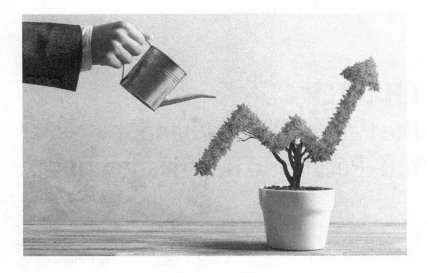

Fig. 4.1 — Growing the practice

"First and foremost, track attrition and reappointment rates," K. Pat Brown, DDS says. "Your reappointment percentage should be at 95% for hygiene."

Your attrition rate is important to track to ensure practice growth. The number of patients coming into the practice should be higher than those leaving or dropping out of your system. To sustain it during times of inflation, and of saturation (new dentists moving into your area), it is imperative to try to keep patients who you already have. Most of those who are not on track with their recommended cleaning schedules are procrastinators, or do not have money, or are short on time. It's not because they do not like you or have gone to another practice.

Your Recall System

Most of your patients just need a gentle nudge to get back on track. One telephone conversation with them about reappointments is usually effective. But what if they don't answer your call? And what if they don't call back when you leave a message? If they're one year or less overdue, you need a system in place to get them back on the books. These patients should be contacted as part of your recall system (Fig. 4.2).

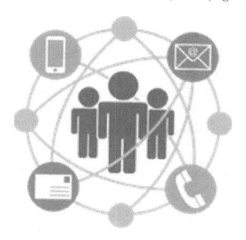

Figure 4.2 — Recall system

Recall Step One–Call overdue patients

The first step is simply running a report of all those patients who were due last month for their hygiene appointments, and contacting them. The front office runs the report, calls everyone on the list, and documents it: Did they leave a message? Did the patient answer and make an appointment? Did they answer and ask not to be called again? Did they have another request that the front office should pay attention to?

Documentation is important so that the patient isn't hounded unnecessarily. We do not want to harass our patients, or make them not want to call us, so pay attention to any special requests. Some practices will run reports and then call the families. Trying people after 4 p.m. is usually best: Between 4 p.m. and 7 p.m. you can often reach a "live body." If a patient is one month overdue for their hygiene appointment, a staff member can make a phone call.

Recall Step Two—Follow up with a postcard, then a letter

If the patient isn't reached by phone, then a month later a postcard can be sent saying that they are missed. At month three, your system should generate a letter saying that they are overdue and explain how important it is for the health of their entire body for them to keep up with oral care.

Recall Step Three—Use an outside service

After three months of not hearing a response from the patient, an outside service can be used. Patient relationship software is utilized to send text messages to your patients not only confirming appointments but also managing overdue patients by sending them messages through text messaging and emails. An outside agency can help with this.

Recall Step Four—Offer free services

At the twelve-month mark, an effective way to encourage a return visit is to offer a free service upon scheduling and coming into the office. Some doctors have offered a free exam and X rays, or free whitening, if the patient returns. Sometimes, even a simple Starbucks gift card will work. If you do this, include a deadline, which will promote action.

Text and Email Communications

You should have a patient relationship partner who can manage patient reviews on social media and who can generate frequent communication between you and your patients with the quick click of a button. A service like this satisfies our culture's need to communicate remotely through text and emails, and it also frees up your staff to have the time to serve your patients in other ways.

Texting and email (Fig. 4.3) have become a social norm. All types of businesses are utilizing these methods to reach their customer base with just a click of a button. It is more efficient, and most patients love the ease of communication; they will think it is cool that you are up to date on the technology.

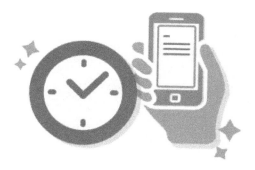

Figure 4.3 — Text and email communication

You can text or email your patient with appointment reminders, which will reduce your no-show or late patient rate. Plus, you can use this software to make reappointments for people who have missed their visits and need to be put back on the books. Contracting with a company that completes confirmations to your patients on your schedule via text reminder or email is, therefore, a valuable time saver. It increases the much-needed patient touch. If patients are thinking about you, they will often promote you.

Now, on to patient reviews. . . . How do you ask for them?

CHAPTER 5
Asking for Patient Reviews: Securing a Five-Star Rating the Ritz-Carlton Way

One of the things I learned during my time with Ritz-Carlton was that personal reviews from satisfied customers are great advertising. In dentistry, reviews—whether by word of mouth or via social media—are necessary for the growth of the practice, and therefore for your hygiene practice-within-the-practice. When you have more patients referring their friends and family, the chairs will naturally stay full. This allows your patients to have a wonderful dental home to go to and it provides a place for great staff to continue their employment and journey to financial prosperity.

Reviews are our "bread and butter" when building a practice, and are the key to having a full schedule. One of the ways to build from within is by straightforwardly asking for reviews (Fig. 5.1). Most of us by nature are not comfortable asking for someone to say nice things about us. But there are a couple of tricks to help you feel comfortable in the approach so you get the reviews you want.

The easiest way to ask for a review is to do it when your patient gives you a compliment. When they say that they love coming to see you and that you give great care for their family, that's a perfect time to ask for them to share their experience with others. I always ask patients to share their experience via Google, Yelp, or with a video testimonial. There are lots of potential patients that would love to hear feedback from current ones, I tell them, and paid advertisements don't tell the real story. Plus, it's expensive to generate a new patient from a paid lead. You get more bang for your buck when you build your practice from within by asking for reviews, and it is more personal.

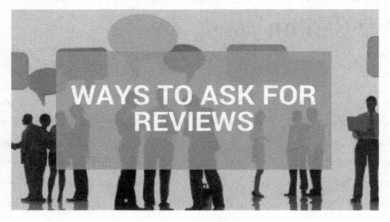

Figure 5.1 — Asking for reviews

Colin Receveur, author of *The Four Horsemen of Dentistry,* writes that it's "more credible . . . when your current patients speak on camera about the experience your future patients can expect with you and your practice. Again, not all videos are created equal. There's an art to getting patient testimonial videos that your prospects can relate to and identify with. That art wasn't covered in your dental school curriculum."

A potential new patient loves to hear that existing patients are receiving great care time and time again (Fig. 5.2). While it may not be in our nature to ask for a compliment, if we express to patients that their review allows us to serve another patient with great care, they won't hold it against us; we need to break out of our comfort zone and just ask.

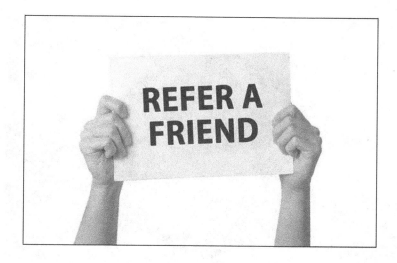

Figure 5.2 — Social networking

People will appreciate knowing that they are going to a great practice when they hear it from a firsthand review—your existing patients. Remember that your existing patients want to please you the way you want to please them. So just ask! Some practices even have an iPad or computer access portal where patients can enter their review right there in the office (Fig. 5.3). That is a great way to ensure that the review gets done. The more reviews you get, the higher up in the search engines you'll go when patients are searching online for a dentist in your area.

So remember, if a patient pays you a compliment, or shares with you how great the front office, assistant, or doctor was, ask for a review! It's the least expensive way to obtain other great patients. As Matthew M. Wasemiller, DDS says, "Doing your best and doing the right thing over and over, day in and day out, is the single best way to grow your practice."

Another way to build your practice with new patients is to ask your existing patients to refer their family and friends to your office.

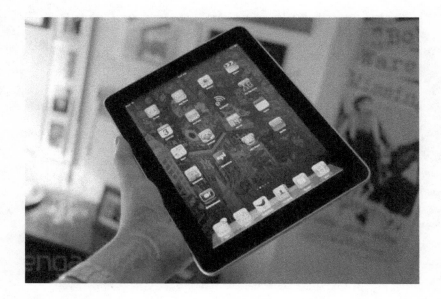

Figure 5.3 — Using an Apple iPad for reviews

Practical Strategies

Colin Receveur, author of *The Four Horsemen of Dentistry*, has a great section in his book called "Survival Strategies" that lays out some principles and practices worth following:

> *Successful dentistry is based on patients liking and trusting you.*
>
> *Prospects won't take your word for it. You have to give them "social proof."*
>
> *Doctor and patient testimonial videos, done well, are an excellent form of social proof.*
>
> *You didn't go to dental school to learn to direct, shoot and edit videos. Outsource them to a reliable company that "gets" dentistry.*
>
> *Online videos and ratings sites are the new word-of-mouth advertising. Managing your online reputation is crucial to your success.*

Once likeability, trust and credibility are established, your practice becomes the only logical choice to solve patients' dental problems.

I would add that you can hang up tastefully-designed posters, or put the request for referrals right on your appointment reminder cards for their next visit.

Being a Hygienepreneur means thinking out of the box to get the "yes" and the "win." Patients naturally think that your practice is busy enough, and won't realize on their own that referrals will help you. Many times I've been paid a compliment by a patient, and said in response, "Please refer your family and friends." Often they respond in a shocked manner: "You're accepting new patients?"

"Of course," I say.

I tell them we are still growing and that we love it when our existing patients refer families and friends because they are amazing people as well. Remember, if you grow your practice, it will support you! Grow your patient base and grow your own schedule. Be in charge of your patient load. If a patient refers a family member to you, they will want to see the hygienist that their friend or family member sees. Your schedule will be full of nice people to take care of, which will both generate more income for the practice and you, and be a pleasant experience!

Online Reviews and Recommendations

On the flip side, it helps to be aware of the referral sources of new patients. Who referred them? If they found you on Yelp (Fig. 5.4), Google, or other online avenues of referral, you want to make sure that their visits always go very smoothly because they're likely to post there themselves.

Do not let things slide when you have a patient in your chair who came by way of Yelp, for instance. While you should always take care of everybody with equal professionalism, make sure that you are on your "A" game when it comes to those folks. As fast as they can give you a good review, they can give you a bad one!

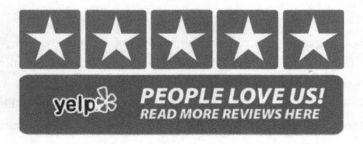

Figure 5.4 —Yelp as a source of referrals

As recently as a couple of decades ago, there were no online reviews. If something bad happened and we had a system failure, we could fix it and smooth it over with the patient and they would be satisfied.

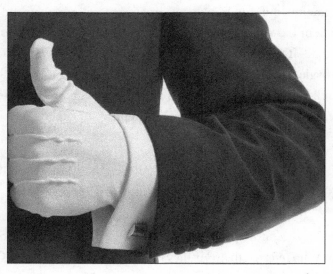

Figure 5.5 — The"white-glove" treatment

Now what happens when Yelpers come to us from an online referral and online review is that they are prompted by Yelp to give feedback about their experience. Even if they had no intention of giving a review, the prompt will remind them to do so and a lot of people who were referred by Yelp will indeed give a review—good or bad. So you want to make sure that when they give a review that it will be good. Be aware of how both new patients and existing patients were referred, and make sure that your customer service level is truly in the "white glove" category (Fig. 5.5).

You might be saying to yourself that you always give five-star service, and everyone you work with is always treated with the optimum care. But we all know that we get busy and sometimes we have system failures. We have the best intentions but we are all human and this happens. We just have to make sure that it never happens to a patient who came to us from an online review source.

We will grow the practice by delivering great service to patients who will give us fantastic reviews. Their reviews will be seen by others who may decide to become patients based on what they read. We all know many of our patients refer friends and family. An online review can serve the same function, but with strangers.

Once you do it, it will be easy. Be more than just a hygiene provider, be a *Hygienepreneur*: Grow your practice and build your level of achievement!

Now, on to adopting a "hospitality" mindset in your dental hygiene career. How do you best do that?

CHAPTER 6
Hygiene and the Practice of Hospitality (Own It and You Retain Your Patients for Life)

As I mentioned in the introduction, my practice foundations stem from my guest hospitality background with La Costa Resort and the Ritz-Carlton. I was trained through an extensive program that encompassed ways of providing "next level" guest services. The "Ritz-Carlton Way" (Fig. 6.1) is a trademarked customer service methodology that I wish all healthcare providers and their teams could learn. As healthcare professionals, we have to treat people better.

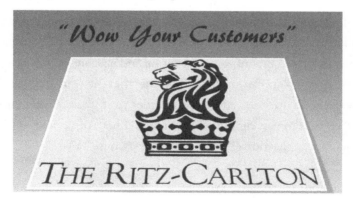

Figure 6.1 — The Ritz-Carlton Way

So, how do you separate yourself from other dental offices? You need to treat the people who come to you as guests, not patients. Provide great healthcare, but do it at a five-star service level that gives your patients (who are your guests) a reason to refer you to other quality patients.

Here are some great ways that you can make your patients feel like they're being treated as they would at a hospitality-focused establishment.

Hospitality = Always Saying "Yes"

I recently had an experience at a wine bar that reminded me of why we need to offer the kind of service you see at a very high-end hotel and golf resort.

The story begins like this: The moment was unscheduled. My fiance and I had stumbled upon this beautiful place and thought that we would eat lunch there, have a glass of wine, and enjoy the beautiful setting amongst all of the trees, fountains, gardens, and birds; Italian music was playing in the background. We were surrounded by Mediterranean architecture and gorgeous stonework that was strategically placed. It was a very spontaneous moment and we were excited to have the new experience. Because the environment was so beautiful and upscale, we just knew that the staff there would be amazing. The way that the wine bar was set up, you could walk up to the counter and order your glass of wine and they would serve it to you right then and there. Then, of course, you could walk to your table yourself. The setting screamed, "Yes!"

The staff communicated, "No."

It was such a disappointment. After ordering my glass of wine, I asked the gentleman for a glass of ice water as well. He told me I couldn't get it there—I would have to walk somewhere else in the bar area to get it. This wasn't a big deal, because it was literally ten feet away, but there was a long line there. So, when I saw how long the line was, I asked if he wouldn't mind just getting me the glass of water since there was a line there and not here. No, he said. I thanked him and went to the other register, where I waited for fifteen minutes (as people ordered drinks) to get a glass of ice water. He continued to not be busy. Unbelievable.

Unfortunately, the negative experience in that beautiful place left me thinking the whole time about him saying "no," and the inconvenience that created. It all happened because their business had a system failure (Fig. 6.2). Why couldn't he get the glass of ice water? Was he not allowed to? Or was it "not his job?" Again, it wasn't about the ice water as much as the impression he gave that he didn't care about me.

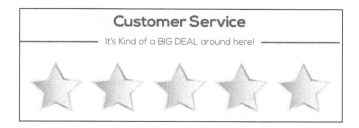

Figure 6.2 — The right service attitude

It's the small things that shape our opinions of businesses we frequent when we walk away from the experience. We have to value our patients' business and make sure that we are handling them with white-glove service, and with no hesitation. They need to see that we want to serve them and say "yes."

The patient is always watching you. Keep that in mind: All actions need to be directed to serving patients' needs. If they see you doing something instead that they perceive as unimportant, they will feel neglected. They should be the number-one focus.

When you are in a service industry, the first answer that should come out of your mouth is "yes" (Fig. 6.3) You need to give customers what they want. You want to satisfy their every need. You want to treat them as a guest, as if you're in your home and they have come by invitation; you want them to accept the invitation and come back.

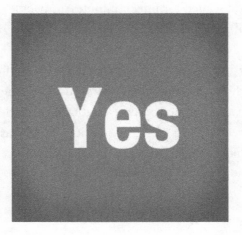

Figure 6.3 — The answer you should aim to give

"Learning how to fulfill each patient's dental desires keeps them coming back," K. Pat Brown, DDS says.

Not all of us have had the opportunity to go to continuing education courses to learn how to be more courteous and how to deliver extra customer service at a level that we've never been trained for. Why not do it? I would recommend that you go to your doctor and ask him to send you to special classes on customer service of the type that the hospitality business is so well known for. It's a great pleasure and honor that patients trust us with their care and their families' care. We have to treat them in a way that shows how honored we are. So explore the options of continuing education in this area. What techniques can you use to help your patients feel like their visit was extra special?

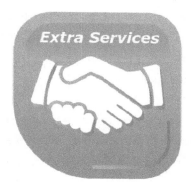

Figure 6.4 — Go the extra mile

Seven Ways to Show Patients They're Valued

Here are some examples from my experience in the dental field which illustrate ways that you can help your patients feel "seen" and valued (Fig. 6.4).

1. ***Remember their personal details***—You will shock your patients if you do this. Most practices do not know the details of their patients' lives. They don't remember if a patient has a new grandbaby on the way, or if a couple planned to go on an Alaskan cruise, or if a younger patient is going to college and will graduate soon. It speaks volumes to your patient when you remember details like this.

    The typical "herding" technique that many hygienists use— where it's all business and all about getting people in and out of the chair— makes people feel like they are just another patient. The greatest tool I ever learned to use was writing notes about my patient's non-dental life in their electronic or physical chart. I write little brief notes based on our conversations in the chair, and then ask the patient about it when they arrive the next time. They are always pleased that I would even remember such details. Every time they come in, I document a new fact to ask about for their next visit.

"The reasoning behind our 'three question rule' and our 'yellow sheets' is to get to know our patients on a deeper level," says Mark A. Costes, DDS. "If they open up to the team or the doctors about important milestones or events in their lives, we always try to capture those comments on our yellow sheets."

Creating that connection helps create trust. That trust ensures that your patient will refer their family and friends. As K. Pat Brown, DDS says, "It is much easier to fish from a stocked pond than a rushing river."

Remember: Patients always feel good when they are treated in a special and unique way.

2. ***Make the day special***—I worked in a practice one time that would hold a "patient appreciation" week during a holiday. This was an awesome concept: They decorated for that holiday and did a huge marketing campaign that showed how much they appreciated their patients.

   You could give them a little gift reflecting the theme of the day, or display signs that you've hung in the practice which recognize that they are loved and valued. These little things add up to more love for you, and patients will go home and tell their family and friends how much they need to go to your office too.

3. ***Why not free Wi-Fi?***—Frequently when I travel, I'll inquire whether there is free Wi-Fi offered (wherever I might be). I'm

not alone: most of us have phones or tablets that we need to connect with. Offering free Wi-Fi to your patients (Fig. 6.5) is a plus, and is easy to set up. Sometimes patients are working while they are waiting to be brought back for a scheduled appointment and need a fast internet connection. They like to check emails, or look at social media updates on Facebook and Instagram. If they have to sit for a minute, it is automatic for folks to jump on their phones to get things done. Having Wi-Fi for them speaks volumes, and shows that you care about their time. You want them to have no hang-ups when they are working. You could print a little sign that says, "We love you and we know you love your Wi-Fi, so here is the secret password." Again, we want patients to feel special. We want them to feel like we have thought about everything to help their visit be more enjoyable; if that includes giving them the Wi-Fi password, well, so be it.

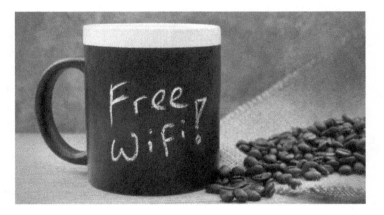

Figure 6.5 — Offer free Wi-Fi

4. **Be "just checking up"**—I personally call patients who received a dental injection from me before I leave for the day to see how they're doing. I call to make sure and to see if they have any questions for me. I finalize the call by telling them how much I appreciate the fact that they continue to choose us for

their care. I tell them that we value them and that I can't wait to see them at their next scheduled appointment.

I have always felt that doctors should be calling their patients too. Most doctors don't do this, in my experience, so when I do see a doctor who does, it always impresses me. I always think, "what a great practice builder!" Check-up calls gains trust, and push the patient forward in telling the world that they have the best dentist on earth (Fig. 6.6). They come in for their next appointment with a positive attitude because they know that the office they have chosen (out of dozens of other offices out there) has their back. They're ready and satisfied, knowing that they chose well.

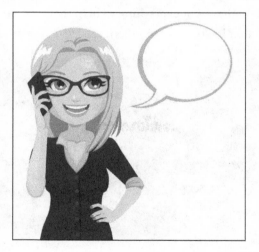

Figure 6.6 — Practice follow-up calls

5. ***Offer refreshments to your patients***—Many years ago, I was very impressed with a practice that I went to for my children's orthodontics. Why? They had an automatic, authentic Starbucks coffee machine (Fig. 6.7) in their beverage service area. They also had a refrigerator that had juice and water available.

Another great idea: Baking bite-size homemade cookies and offering those to your patients—it makes the office smell good. Offering a little hot cocoa, tea, or coffee makes the atmosphere more like the lobby of a high-end hotel than a dental office. It's operating at that "next level" that will separate your practice from others.

The front office should always act as a concierge to the practice. Offering the amenities of the practice and encouraging patient guests access to all those amenities is everything. Again, we need to create comfort. We need to create a level of appreciation that surpasses anything that patient has ever experienced. Remember, patients do not grade their dentist based upon how perfect a margin might be on crowned molar. They grade how good their dentist is based upon how they are treated and how they feel when they leave.

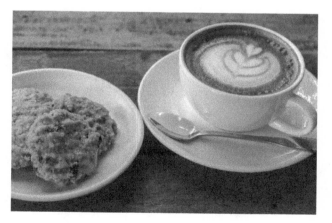

Figure 6.7 — Make refreshments available

I once attended a dental seminar where a speaker said that she had worked for a doctor who was, in her opinion, just "fair" in his skill level. She only worked with him for a short time, but what was interesting was that his patients always said how great a dentist he was. His filling and crown margins weren't perfect, although they were sealed well, but he was nice, courteous, and his chair-side manner was so fantastic that the patients thought that he really was the best dentist in the world, and that his staff was the best staff in the world. This was all because that office had a niche: They knew how to treat people with white-glove service and did it in a way that was consistent and excellent. That practice grew 100% by offering superior hospitality and by just being really friendly to everyone (Fig. 6.8).

I always loved that story. What she spoke about was so true. I have gone to restaurants and ordered a meal that ended up being just average in quality but have enjoyed it more because of how I was treated. We can't forget that patients have lots of choices. We have to continue to separate ourselves from the others and evolve and say "yes" as often as we can.

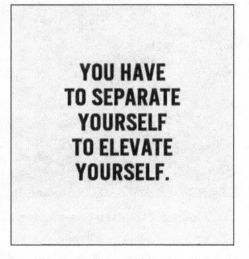

**YOU HAVE
TO SEPARATE
YOURSELF
TO ELEVATE
YOURSELF.**

Figure 6.8— Words to live by

6. ***Help your patients relax***—Our senses are very important. What we see, smell and hear helps us formulate an opinion

about our environment. As such, we need to make sure that our dental offices have soothing music playing in the background, music that is universally enjoyed (Fig. 6.9). We need to make sure that the colors on the inside of the practice are very warm and comforting. And it is important for our reception areas and common areas to be really clean. All of that speaks volumes to the patient, who otherwise might worry about how clean our dental instruments and tools are.

The goal is to increase the experience of relaxation. The lighting should be right, and be sure to offer patients headphones so that they can listen to their music instead of hearing the suctions, drills, and sterilization equipment. That's another reason to give them the Wi-Fi password, so they can listen with their own headphones on their own phone.

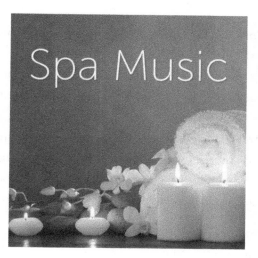

Figure 6.9 — Appropriate music helps patients relax

Don't overlook scents, either. All-natural aromatherapy, either inserted in the AC vents or in portable units, adds further ambience to the practice. The Mandalay Bay Hotel in Las Vegas used to have an elite section of the hotel called "The Hotel at the Mandalay." Every single time we went into that portion of the hotel you would smell something different in the air—lavender one day, oranges the next, gardenias after that. It was an amazing addition to the luxurious setting of this hotel. I always felt that dental offices should do that too. It really does make the environment more relaxing and more pleasant.

Sometimes dental offices can be chilly. Offering sterile blankets and little pillows that the patient can take home with them is an awesome idea, right? How about warm, scented hand towels presented after a patient appointment to help the patient freshen up and feel clean after their long procedure? While our fees have to reflect the cost of such extras, they're so worth it because they speak volumes about the quality of care we give.

7. ***Start with a smile***—The biggest form of hospitality doesn't cost a dime. Just being very courteous, nice, and helpful, with a big smile, is so important. It all starts with a smile and the notion that "I need to serve." Giving our patients compliments and telling them how much we like them and appreciate them is huge and will not go unnoticed. We should be excited about the care that they are going to receive and that they have received. By showing them "before" and "after" pictures, and by genuinely being excited about their care, we will get them excited as well.

Now, how about hygiene handoffs to other team members? What are the best strategies?

CHAPTER 7
Hygiene Handoffs to Other Team Members

Communication with patients is a key component of success, but so is communication among team members. When a team is communicating well, patients see it and gain confidence that they've chosen the right practice.

Good communication skills are learned and should be practiced. Flow and timing are also important. I have always promoted the "hand-off" technique, which I'll explain below. This skill, when done well, is amazing and leaves everyone feeling confident because they know that a message is being heard and understood. Patient care increases and workplace stress decreases because the practice is operating at a higher level of patient care. Handoffs are crucial to making the patient's experience great, and to team building.

In an ideal practice, our team members are in the business of patient care. We want to do this in the best way, so that we feel a sense of pride. The handoff is the key to making it happen. When done right, hygienist and dentist are fluid and well-rehearsed, and their jobs are easier to do; meanwhile, patients sit smiling in their chairs, knowing that they are being taken care of. They are our number one focus. They are the reason we do what we do, and it shows. So, communicate and practice the handoff. Show your patients that all team members know what the plan is, then drive it.

What Is a "Handoff"?

In a football offense, one player takes the football and then hands it off to another player to advance and score. We do much the same thing in dentistry, all day long. The transition of the patient from one team member to another is always smoother with a proper handoff. When the two team members communicate well together, it also raises the confidence of the patient about the practice. People always like to be talked about when it's something complimentary, right?

During a handoff, two staff members should enthusiastically share information in front of the patient in a three-way conversation that helps make the patient feel valued and cared for, and shows that any concerns were heard and addressed. This type of communication reduces miscommunication between team members and patients. If the patient wants to update any concerns, the handoff is the time to verify the patient's requests and needs.

There are five handoffs that the hygienist can engage in:

1. Dentist to hygienist for a new patient
2. Dental assistant to hygienist
3. Hygienist to dental assistant
4. Hygienist to dentist
5. Hygienist to front office

Let's look at each of them.

1. Dentist to Hygienist: New Patient

Here's a possible script the dentist could use for this handoff:

DENTIST: "Hi, Amber. Mrs. Jones is all ready for you. Mrs. Jones, this is Amber, our fantastic hygienist. We were able to come up with a plan together. She has a few areas of concern that we will address. The upper right tooth has decay at the margin of the existing crown that is over ten years old and will need a new crown. We were also able to evaluate her gum tissue. She has had periodontal treatments in the past but it has been a while since her last cleaning. She needs more visits with you to do scaling and root planing to remove the debris under the gumline. I did discuss laser therapy with her as well to help combat the inflammation that you will see. We think a three-month recall will also be advisable. If you could discuss good tools for her at home, that would be awesome. Okay, Mrs. Jones, if you don't have any more questions for me, I will leave you with Amber. She will take great care of you."

2. Dental Assistant to Hygienist

The assistant handoff to the hygienist usually occurs when a patient is seeing the doctor for treatment or for an exam. In this handoff, the dental assistant usually escorts the patient to the hygiene room, where the handoff will take place. Sometimes the hygienist will see the patient in another room where they have been getting another procedure done, and the dental assistant will deliver to the hygienist facts about the patient using the patient's name, then provide additional information about the patient, including what procedures were completed for the patient that day, and say something nice, like, "it went well." One of the team members should be sure to ask whether the patient needs another appointment with the doctor.

It's also valuable for the dental assistant to tell the hygienist, in front of the patient, what comes next. The patient is then guided through the dental experience and is made aware that every team member in the office knows what is on the care plan. A proper handoff achieves two things. First, it reassures patients that their visit was a positive one that went well and that they made the right decision in showing up and having the work completed. And second, it promotes to patients the idea that everyone is on the same page with regard to what's next on the agenda, and that the team is there to guide them through it. Either way, like a relay team on a track (Fig. 7.1), responsibility for the patient should be handed off gently, like a baton being passed from one team member to the next.

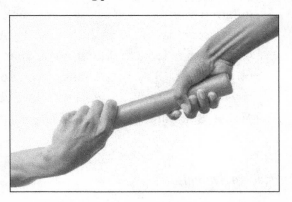

Figure 7.1 — The handoff

Here is an example of what it might sound like:

DENTAL ASSISTANT: "Hi Shalon, this is Jon. Jon, Shalon is going to be taking care of all of your hygiene concerns.

Shalon, Jon just had the best exam with Dr. Brown. He had all of his images completed, and he and the doctor discussed a plan to start on the upper right of his mouth. Dr. Brown would like an hour to work on those two teeth and will work on the lower left of the mouth after that. Jon, do you have any questions for me or Dr. Brown?"

If the patient doesn't have any questions, simply say, "Okay, good! Shalon is going to take great care of you. Thank you, Shalon!"

If it is a new patient, a full introduction between the patient and hygienist should be given, but if it is an existing patient, the assistant can just say the patient's name. Saying someone's name in front of them, or to them, increases value and trust.

Here's an example of a situation where the patient has just had a treatment procedure with the doctor and now has an appointment with the hygienist:

DENTAL ASSISTANT: "Hi Julie! Our great patient, Jon, here had the best appointment today with the doctor. He had his two fillings and crown completed on the upper right of his mouth. We just need to see him back in two weeks to finish and deliver the permanent crown. We can treat the lower right at the same time to save Jon a visit. We just need two hours reserved.

Okay Jon, you are in great hands here with Julie, and we will see you next time. Thank you, Julie! Jon, have a great day!"

The patient should be delivered with care, in a short but sweet manner. There's no need for a long-winded handoff. Time management should always be recognized so that you continue to stay on time throughout the day. Using a methodical approach in a handoff ensures efficiency. Do it every time to aleviate miscommunication and promote increased patient retention and acceptance.

3. Hygienist to Dental Assistant

If the doctor will be seeing the patient after the hygienist, it is good to pre-communicate with the staff where the patient will be taken next. When the staff is ready and prepared for the next step, it shows the patient that the team rocks! You want to operate like a smoothly running machine. Convey this information to all team members in advance, so when you escort the patient to the designated treatment room, there is no miscommunication. Patients do not need to know that you and the assistant have already discussed maneuvering them from one room to the next. It is just done smoothly. You need to promote five-star service (Fig. 7.2). When you care for your patients in a "white glove" manner, you will get superb results.

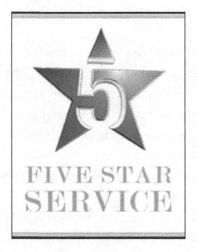

Figure 7.2 — Five-star service

Everyone needs to be "on point," and the preparation needs to be in place to ensure flawless execution and fantastic results. After all, we are always "on stage," in a sense. Practice makes perfect, and you need to develop excellent communication skills to help manage every concern your patients have. The skill of communication via the handoff technique can give great results when used to its fullest.

Here is an example of a hygienist handing a patient off to the assistant:

HYGIENIST: "Hi Brandi, this is our patient, Chris. Chris, Brandi is one of the doctor's dental assistants and is going to take great care of you with Dr. Brown today. Chris just had a nice visit. He had all of his images completed and we cleaned his teeth, checked his gums, and he is scheduled back for his next hygiene appointment in six months. Chris did have a question regarding whether he was a good candidate for Invisalign, and he was also concerned about the shape of his front tooth. He may want to have a cosmetic consultation regarding that. His health history is good and there are no changes since we saw him last. Have I covered everything, Chris?"

You can then say to Chris, "Brandi and Dr. Brown are going to take great care of you. I look forward to seeing you next time. Thank you, Brandi!"

4. Hygienist to Dentist

What are our doctors' goals when they enter our operatory? Well, you know that they are very busy juggling their own procedures in their own operatories, all while trying to also satisfy all of the exams that come out of hygiene. It doesn't matter if there is one hygienist or multiple hygienists, all needing exams—the time our doctors have is extremely limited. It is easier if there are multiple doctors to help ease the load of the schedule.

However, if there is just one doctor, then the hygienists have to be sensitive and respectful of his or her time. We need to have a plan and a strategy to help our doctors fulfill all of the needs of our patients for their exams, but in a timely fashion that is efficient and straightforward. So, when the doctor comes into the operatory, we need to have that patient ready.

Doing a handoff helps deliver information in a thorough and efficient manner that helps everyone. It should be well scripted, not leaving out any details, to ensure that the doctor gets all of the information. That way, his exam is comprehensive and the patient feels satisfied that the care was excellent.

There are four steps with a "Hygiene to Doctor" handoff:

STEP 1: When the doctor comes in the operatory, make sure you say the patient's name; that way, the doctor does not have to look at a chart to remember who they are. Say the patient's name in this way: "Oh, thank you, Dr. Jones, for coming in to see Sheila for her exam today." Making sure to say the patient's name is a great tool for everybody. We always want patients feeling that their doctor remembers them.

STEP 2: Provide a quick personal update about the patient. For example, you can share with the doctor that Sheila is expecting another grandchild and that they are waiting to get the call from their daughter anytime with the news of the upcoming arrival. Saying something personal helps the patient feel at ease and helps promote trust and a friendly environment (Fig. 7.3).

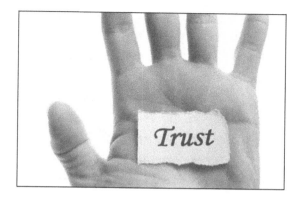

Figure 7.3 — The importance of trust

Personal contact shows patients that you care not only about their dental health, but about what is going on in their lives as well. This always makes for a great impression.

STEP 3: Provide a brief update about the patient's clinical issues. Be sure to include any existing treatment recommendations that are on the list. You can also share any medical updates, whether there are changes or not.

STEP 4: Provide a brief periodontal health update. Let your doctor know what recall you have them scheduled for to maintain the bone and tissue level. Also, let the doctor know how the periodontal exam went, and the state of the patient's home care. The doctor can then start the exam.

Here is another example of what you can say:

HYGIENIST: "Dr. Jones, thank you so much for coming in to see Sheila today. She's doing so good! She and her husband are expecting their fifth grandchild, so everybody is on baby watch. It's so great that she's here with us today. Sheila said that her teeth feel fantastic and there are no issues to report. Also, since her last exam, there are no current treatment needs or recommendations. We do keep Sheila on a three-month recall to maintain her bone level, and she's doing really good with her home care."

At that point, the doctor can exchange niceties with Sheila about the grandbaby coming, and then do the exam and move on.

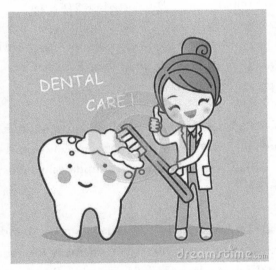

Figure 7.4 — A positive attitude

The doctor should be in and out of your room in less than ten minutes. Be sure to have all of the images up for the doctor, which will help with time management. The biggest part of doing a handoff is to always stay positive as you deliver the message (Fig. 7.4). We always want our patients to feel that they are doing a good job, and that we appreciate their efforts. If they need to focus on a particular area, for example, we can let them know that we understand how hard it is to reach that area, but if they try a certain angle maybe they will find it to be easier.

Patients want to have a dental team that is supportive and positive. They do not want to go to an office or see a hygienist who is negative, or who will lecture them. So, as healthcare providers, we need to find a way to deliver the message in a positive, supportive, caring way that will make the patient feel that we understand their challenges and are there to help them.

Mike Czubiak, DDS and Steve Sperry put it this way:

> *Confidence comes from believing in yourself, your industry and the science. Confidence is situational. Confidence becomes influential when you believe. Do you believe? How much bleeding on probing is acceptable? You know this. . . . Do you believe it? I don't want to sound dated but the character, Stuart Smalley (from the TV show, SNL), was known to say "I am good enough, I am smart enough, and doggone it, people like me." That was his mantra for success. I believe in you.*

5. Hygienist to Front Office

Our front office staff are great multitaskers. They see a lot of people coming in and out of the office during the day. They handle all of the providers of the practice as well as all of the patients that come in. So it is important for us to help our front office with their time since they have so little of it. The handoff shortens timetables for checking out a patient, and also reduces the risks of miscommunication. Hitting on the key points of interest, while delivering that patient to the front office, is the last step of their visit that day. It is a streamlined process, but it is extremely important. It should be said the same way, every single time you bring up a patient.

There are three crucial pieces of information that your front office wants to know:

STEP 1: Say the patient's name. Say the patient had a nice visit. Also, tell the front office staff that you have already scheduled the patient's hygiene appointment.

STEP 2: Did you do as scheduled for that appointment, or did the schedule change that day? Or did some procedure need to be modified?

STEP 3: Did your patient have any treatment needs after seeing the doctor for an exam today? If there was no exam with the doctor that day, but the patient has some treatment to take care of, make sure to bring it up to the front office that these needs are recommended and the doctor would like "X amount" of time for the next visit.

An example of a good handoff would sound like this:

HYGIENIST: "Hi Wendy! Lisa, Wendy is our treatment sched-
                uling coordinator. Lisa had a great visit today. We
                went ahead and did the exam as scheduled, and
                we have already scheduled her back for her next
                hygiene appointment. She does need to come
                back to see Dr. Brown for the lower left tooth and
                it would be great if you could help us coordinate
                a time that is good for both Lisa and the doctor.
                Lisa, Wendy is going to take great care of you! We
                look forward to seeing you next time. Thank you,
                Wendy."

The hygienist should leave at that point so the treatment coordinator can present the information to the patient with no interruptions.

Remember, making sure to do the handoff the same way every time will streamline your system and will help you and your team every time with time management too. Everyone will be happy because everyone will be on time!

That leads us to the hygiene experience for your existing patients. What are the best practices?

CHAPTER 8
The Hygiene Experience for Existing Patients

Make sure that your game face is always on for your existing patients, just as it is for new patients.

Remember, veteran patients never want to feel that we've let our level of customer service fall just because they are familiar, like family. We actually want to treat them *better than family*! They are our true voices in the referral game, the patients who truly have experienced our practice and have seen us in different contexts. Let's not forget this. We need to always be game-day ready, whether for a new patient or existing patient. The stage is always bright, and the mics are on!

New patients get a lot of attention, and everyone naturally focuses on them: how to market to a new patient, how much that new patient is worth based upon how much it costs to get them into your practice, how much diagnosis comes out of a new patient exam that is comprehensive, and so forth. All of these factors are extremely important. However, the existing patient, over time, is of even greater value.

Although we always want to treat patients as valued individuals, and care for them according to the highest ethical and professional standards, from a business standpoint it sometimes helps to look at them in terms of a dollar amount (Fig. 8.1).

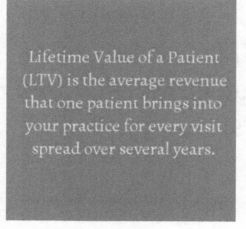

Figure 8.1 — Lifetime value of a patient
(Years x Visits x Average Fee = Value)

Consider how much that patient is going to spend in your practice every year on average in their lifetime. The industry standard is that the lifetime value of a patient can be calculated by counting how many years the patient has been coming to your practice, multiplied by how many times a year they are seen in your office, and then by the average fee that they pay per visit.

This value should give you a dollar amount that shows the patient's "net worth" to the practice. Mark A. Costes, DDS, who is CEO of the Dental Success Institute, calculates the patient's dollar value based upon a twenty-year term. If you were going to practice for twenty years, and were lucky enough to retain that patient for the same amount of time, and the patient averaged two visits a year, then that patient would be worth $125 at each visit, he calculates. Dr. Costes states that this number is conservative, but based upon average hygiene goals.

Most practices operate above $125 per visit, but to keep it conservative we could use that number and calculate from that the average. So if the patient pays $250 each year x twenty years, then the whole dollar amount earned by the office would be $5,000. If the patient averages one restorative dental procedure, like broken tooth repair or a cusp that needs a crown, and that procedure happens once every four years at $1,000, then the patient's net worth becomes $9,000, according to Dr. Costes' calculations.

Dr. Costes does not stop there when calculating the value of one patient. If that patient likes you and you keep him or her happy, this too is a huge source of additional revenue. If the patient refers friends and family at a conservative rate of one per every five years, and those visits produce $9,000 as well, then that original patient is worth not $9,000 but $45,000! That number is super exciting, and a great reason why existing patients need to be given white-glove service every time to keep them coming in and doing good things to help your practice grow.

So let's get started on how best to make that existing patient experience exceptional. It all starts with the greeting.

You need to greet patients like your team has been waiting for them all day! Say hello to them like they are a friend visiting from out of town who has just arrived by plane (Fig. 8.2). When you walk out to the reception area, say hello, and genuinely greet that patient with a big smile, it speaks volumes.

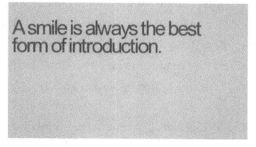

Figure 8.2 — Introductions

Also let the patient know that you appreciate them coming in for their visit today. Show that you know how busy they are and that you appreciate them fitting you into their schedule.

When we take that attitude, it makes them feel appreciated and valued. The white-glove service (Fig. 8.3) where we accept that patient for their appointment with our team is crucial.

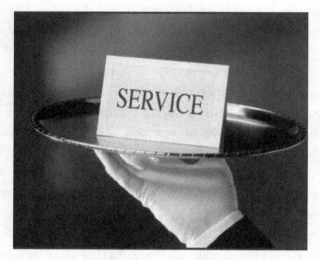

Figure 8.3 — Greeting existing patients with white-glove service

Each patient needs to be treated as if no others have been seen that day, or will be seen that day: it is all about this visit. After you greet your patients and escort them back to your operatory, invite them to take a seat and ask if you can hang their coat for them, or put their bags and phone in a safe place. After they are settled and comfortable in your chair, then you can ask them how their family is and how they are doing. Remember, you're there to serve them. You don't know what kind of day they've had or what they are up against next, all you know is that while they are in your office, you're going to put their mind at ease knowing that they will get the great care that they deserve, with great service at an exceptional value. They should leave that office feeling secure that they made the right choice in coming to you.

Most practices that I've been to do a great job of writing some personal notes about their patients' last visits. The patients are always amazed when they think that we've remembered the cruise they were going on, the grandbaby that was due to be born, or the child that was graduating and going off to college. Although we've reminded ourselves with notes, the point is that we appear to have remembered spontaneously, which shows them that we care. So, feel free to make notes in the patient's chart; it will help you and your team stay on a personal level with your patients. You will join their "circle of trust" because you've cared enough to remember what has been going on in their lives. They will feel like they "belong."

The next step is to ask the patient if there are any health changes and how their teeth and gums are feeling today. It is also good to ask if there is anything you can share with the doctor on their behalf.

Take note of this. That way, when the doctor comes in, you can relay the message, which will save patients from having to repeat themselves. Then we ask permission to perform the procedures that are scheduled. Asking the patient permission to proceed shows respect, and it adds a sense of teamwork to their dental care. That way, they are also involved in their own healthcare. It is their teeth and gums and overall health that you are taking care of, so of course, the patient is in charge.

It makes patients feel very good to know that your level of service is given based upon their needs. While completing their dental care, check in with your patients to make sure they are feeling good and are comfortable.

Sometimes, as hygienists, we get focused on the task at hand and forget that we have a patient in the chair who may be nervous, and who would definitely like to be somewhere else. If we ask them how they are feeling and how they are doing, it brings us back to why we are doing what we are doing—we are there every day seeing patients because we care about people. When patients know that you care about how they were feeling during the visit, and making sure that they are not feeling any discomfort, they're likely to come back for another visit.

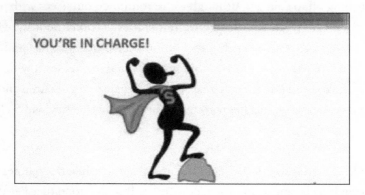

Figure 8.4 — Recruiting the patient for the team

This has always been very important to me when I "temp" in an office. The number-one job of a temporary hygienist, or a temporary provider, is to not hurt the patient in the chair. You want that patient leaving with no complaints, and scheduling another visit that they will show up for because they had a great experience. We need to remember as providers that we are in the service industry, even though we are technically healthcare providers. Each patient should be treated as a guest who you want returning for another visit. You want them to be happy, and the goal should be to make them so happy that they will refer family and friends to you.

"Never stop wowing and educating your patients," says K. Pat Brown, DDS.

After the clinical part of their visit is done, sit the patient up in the chair and say thank-you for coming in for the day, and that you hope that the visit was a good one. Then, wait for it.

What are you waiting for? You're waiting for the compliment that is going to come from them on a job well done. That's the moment when you can ask for a review from them.

Unlike the new patient, you have already established a long-term relationship with returning patients, and they trust you. When you ask for a review, you will most likely get a "yes." Escort the patient to the front after making their next appointment. Do a fantastic handoff to your front office, thank the patient again by name for coming in, and thank your front office staff for taking great care of your patient. And then do it all again.

I cannot stress enough how important existing patients are, both to building our practices and to completing our mission as hygienists of providing help to others—a mission that allows us to take care of our own families as well. Using the right words to explain what we do helps your patients, new or existing, have confidence in you and the care that you give. You, in turn, have more confidence when you know what you are talking about, and that shows through to the patient.

So, what about really getting to know your patients on a personal level? Everyone is different, and we need to cater to those differences to provide a unique experience. Let's analyze it in Chapter 9 . . . .

CHAPTER 9
Knowing Your Patient to Gain a Trusted Partner

Whether it is a new patient or an existing patient, one of the biggest challenges in our profession is "reading" what type of patient you have in your chair. Being able to read your patients' motivations is a skill that all of us should develop.

The first thing we need to do is listen to our patients. We need to listen to what their concerns are, what drives them, and what their motivations are. We also need to understand their backgrounds and their past history. We really have to become very good listeners and watchers.

Reading people doesn't always come naturally—it is a learned skill. Personally, I have gone to many seminars and continuing education classes about communication, and listening skills (Fig. 9.1) are often a big part of what's taught.

I have been so thankful to be able to go to those courses. If you can't attend one, books and seminars out there address how to learn the techniques. Practicing them until they become skills is key. But it all starts with listening.

You should list motivating factors in every patient's chart during your assessments. Getting to know your patient helps you take care of them better. The patient is satisfied when the needs that they consider most important are met. So let's make sure we pay attention and listen to our patients, even if it means straightforwardly asking your patient what's important to them and what their dental goals might be. It's *okay* to ask! The fact that you're even asking speaks volumes.

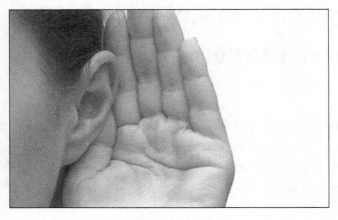

Figure 9.1 — Listening to the patient

Unfortunately, most practices do not ask their patients what they want and what they think they need, which can get things started on the wrong foot. Remember that we are in a partnership with our patients where that patient's dental management is concerned. As hygienists, we're there to guide them in the decision-making about the process of their care, and then delivering that care. In doing so, we want to make sure to meet and exceed their expectations. To do that we have to be good listeners—we have to take the time to sit back and just open our ears.

Matthew M. Wasemiller, DDS sums it up this way: "Always take care of patients' needs first and foremost, focusing on their best interests, and everything else will fall into place."

The Importance of Communication for the Hygienepreneur

When I started writing this book over twos year ago, my goal was to make every hygienist's professional dreams come true. I wanted all hygienists to be able to practice more efficiently with less stress and fatigue, and be entrepreneurs within their dental practice (Fig. 9.2). I wanted them to be able to self-start and lead a movement of dental hygienists who deliver great patient care every day, and who build their practices by taking leading roles as Hygienepreneurs.

It really starts with us genuinely wanting to deliver great health services to our patients. We have to think about making sure that we are practicing in a smart way and doing business intelligently. Communication is key when it comes to making sure that we get a "yes" from our patients, every time. So let's take the time and get to know our patients, give them the service they deserve, and build the practice to success!

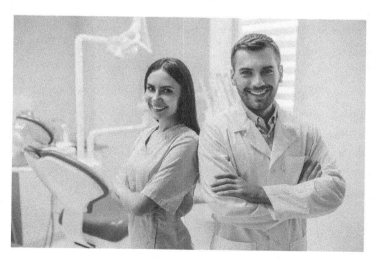

Figure 9.2 — The care team

Making sure we get to know the patient's background and what emotions and events they associate with their dental history is necessary in evaluating where the patient's goals for care and readiness lie. What are their motivations? What events occurred or are going to occur that will affect their course of action?

For example, if the patient has had a poor experience in the past in a dental practice, we need to know this and make sure not to repeat what bothered them. All patients' needs are different, as are their motivating factors. Some may have a family history or event that we need to know about to formulate what really matters to them. For instance, if a patient shares with you that his mother lost her teeth at a young age, and it bothers him, you need to make sure to continue to reassure the patient that you will do everything in your power with their partnership to save his teeth.

Again, ask questions and listen. Let patients know that you want for them what they want for themselves. Learn this skill and you will have a patient for life! You'll be able to fill your chair with happy patients who are a pleasure to see. Life will be easier for you, and for them, simply because you just listened.

After you've filled the seats, you have to work on the task of keeping them filled by being in charge and operating in a smart way. Doing your job in its entirety ensures a full schedule that is productive, and the level of your patient care will be amazing—all because you worked hard, and it shows.

Now it's on to Part III, and how to avoid scheduling problems.

III. SCHEDULING TECHNIQUES TO SAVE THE DAY

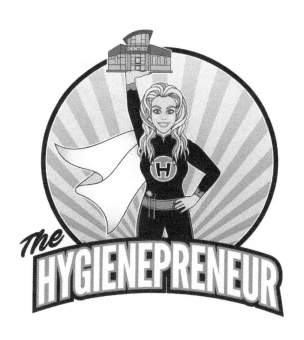

CHAPTER 10
Managing Your Schedule and Taking Control of Your Production

Be savvy when it comes to your schedule. It is your bible and should be handled with care, messaged, and managed, because it's all yours. There are many examples on how to accomplish this.

If your patients need a hygiene appointment for six months later, make sure to enter all of the necessary treatment for that visit into your schedule. Note whether X rays will be done that day, or fluoride treatment, or anything else. Knowing what the patient needs and noting their insurance benefits is a huge bonus to scheduling for success and to meet your productivity goals.

Most hygienists don't know what insurance benefits the patient is eligible for. That needs to change. Be sure to ask your front office to pre-screen all patient insurance benefits and pass the information on to you, including fluoride benefits, frequency on X rays, sealant benefits, frequencies for children, scaling and root planing (SRP) benefits and frequency, prophy and perio maintenance therapy benefits and frequency, and benefits for desensitizing a tooth. Having this information, you could possibly do additional procedures on the same day that you perform their cleaning, and do it all in a more timely fashion.

Time management is crucial when it comes to hygiene productivity. If the front office already has gathered this data, then you can quote it to the patient and perform it in just minutes based on what is in the system. It is important for you, as the hygienist, to become savvy when it comes to procedures and insurance, but you will need the help of your front office. This is critical in becoming a Hygienepreneur.

Dictating adjuncts and pretreatment planning, and the implementation of the care in a timely manner, is very important to patient health and to the financial success of the practice. After all of the hygiene appointments are made with the correct procedures attached from the treatment plan guide, walk the patient to the front office and do your handoff to the administrator.

The handoff (*see Chapter 7*) is super important when delivering the patient to the front office team. Your front office staff should be ready to accept that patient from you as you start to debrief them on the visit that just happened. Greet your front office team member and say hello to them, then tell them that your patient "had a great visit today." Make sure to use the patient's first name. When you use their name while talking to other team members, or to the patient, it creates value: patients feels like they matter to you because you used their names. They feel important and pampered.

Here is an example:

HYGIENIST: "Hi Wendy! Annmarie had a great visit today. We did the exam as scheduled and she and the doctor have come up with a fantastic plan together. We went ahead and scheduled her back for four quadrants of SRP, disinfection with the laser, and fluoride to help areas where roots are exposed. She still needs an appointment with the doctor, so I shared with her that you are an expert at managing the doctor's schedule. If you could help us with that, it would be amazing. The doctor needs an hour and a half with her at the next visit starting with the upper right quadrant."

And then you would say to the patient:

"Annmarie, it was fantastic meeting you! Wendy is going to take great care of you and I can't wait to see you next time! Thank you so much, Wendy."

This handoff is crucial and necessary to complete every single time, with every patient. Your front office needs your help and direction. What's more, when the office team exhibits good communication with the care team, it gives the patient a sense of security and shows them that they are in good hands and will be taken care of every time.

If you did not do work that was scheduled with the patient, then make sure you share that information with your front office and let them know that you updated the computer schedule to show the changes. If there is a routing slip or routing note involved, make sure to change it as well. New patients usually should have more time scheduled for their visit. However, not every patient takes the same amount of time to see. Tailoring the schedule to fit your patients' needs is more productive and improves patient care.

Now, let's discuss making last-minute changes to your hygiene schedule. . . .

CHAPTER 11
Making Last Minute Changes to Your Hygiene Schedule: Pre-plan and Fill it Up

Your goal should be to protect your schedule, and to create the perfect schedule for you. Every day should begin with a morning huddle, in which schedules are discussed.

The morning huddle is invaluable. Spending ten minutes evaluating today's and tomorrow's schedule is crucial to maximizing productivity.

If a patient calls on the same day as their reserved hygiene appointment and tries to cancel, the front office should make every effort to prevent this from happening (Fig. 11.1). Gently ask the patient if there is any way to still come in.

You or the front desk team member might explain to the patient like this:

FRONT OFFICE: "Your hygienist has reserved that time for you, She was looking forward to seeing you. If there's any way you can make it, we would really appreciate it."

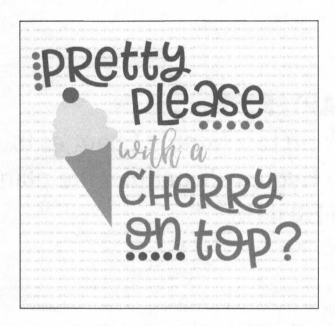

Figure 11.1 — Politely ask that patients keep their appointments

Don't use this language if the patient is ill or has a family emergency, though. Wish them well and get them rescheduled for another day. As a side note, the proper language should be like this:

FRONT OFFICE: "Jerry, I'm so sorry to hear that you are ill. We hope that you feel better, and I will tell Sally that you are unable to come in today. Her schedule is really full, though, so let's go ahead and get you rescheduled for another date and time when you are feeling better."

We should never ask the patient *if* they want to reschedule, or tell them to "just call us back." These are scheduling taboos. Make every effort to get them reappointed. Remember, we are managing the attrition rate, and the words we use matter (Fig. 11.2). In order to do so, what we say needs to be on point.

We should never ask permission to schedule the next appointment, just politely tell them we are going to do so. Nine times out of ten, they will agree and let us guide them into another appointment reservation. Then we need to get cracking to fill that hole!

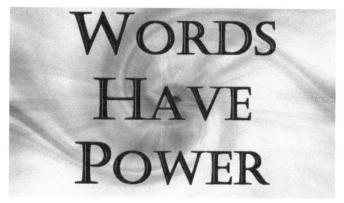

Figure 11.2 — Choosing your words carefully

Short Call List

Using a short call list to fill this time is a lifesaver. This list needs to be built up over time so it can "save the day" for later use.

How do we build that list? It's easy. If the front office receives a call from another patient who is overdue after their appointment was made, the front office scheduler should ask that patient if he or she would like to be called in sooner if a time comes available. When the patient says yes, their name can be added to the "short call" list.

Gary Kadi, author of *Million Dollar Dentistry,* offers this advice: "Keep a short call list or a wish list handy for your appointment coordinator. These are individuals who would be happy to come in on a given day and time, if such appointments open up. That way, if those slots suddenly open, you've got people on the short call list who can fill them immediately."

This list can be accessed and updated using dental management software. Every popular program includes this functionality, and it can be customized for the practice's needs.

Piggybacking on the Dentist's Schedule

The second way the schedule can be filled with ease is by looking at the existing schedule on the doctor's side and seeing if anyone needs a hygiene appointment. A lot of times patients love it when we save them from having to come in again by "piggybacking" appointments. The hygienist can see them before or after the doctor's appointment. If it is an open time that will work before or after the dental appointment, call the patient and say something like this:

FRONT OFFICE: "Mrs. Jones, I wanted to call you right away. A last minute, unexpected change occurred with Angela's schedule that allows for you to get your teeth cleaned right before the doctor sees you today. Would you like to take advantage of this change? It will save you from having to come back."

This usually works really well because most people have reserved time in their schedule for the dental appointment anyway, so what is an extra forty-five minutes or an hour?

Also, if that same patient has a family member who is due or overdue for an appointment that they can bring in with them, even better. That family member can have their hygiene appointment at the same time as the patient's doctor appointment. Making it convenient and easy for families is important, but we sometimes need to think for them, managing their dental care and their appointments. If we help them with this, they will appreciate us more, and our schedules will stay full.

Looking a Week Ahead

The third way an open time slot can be filled is by looking ahead at the same time next week and moving patients forward. As an example, the language would be like this:

FRONT OFFICE: "Mrs. Smith, our hygienist, Angela, had a last-minute change to her schedule today, and she thought of you. Would it be more convenient for you to come in today for your hygiene appointment instead of next week?"

If the patient says yes, we tell her, "great, I will let Angela know; we look forward to seeing you today at 1:00pm instead of next week."

One word of caution: Before pulling forward from the schedule, be sure to check on insurance involvement to review date guidelines. We don't want to bring patients in early and have the insurance company refuse to pay for the bill because it does not fall within their date parameters.

Check Your Lists

The last resort is to utilize our "broken appointment" lists, recall lists, and the hygienists' personal list of people who may want to come in for an appointment. We should leave no stone unturned (Fig. 11.3). As hygienists, we must learn to be involved and make calls ourselves. We can't always rely on our front desk staff to help fill the schedule.

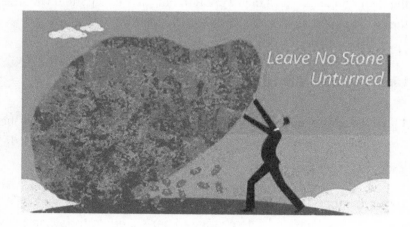

Figure 11.3 — Persistence pays off

No-show and cancellation rates should be traced. When this number climbs towards ten percent, the practice (and you) will experience severe revenue losses. Your efforts toward filling those holes will be rewarded with a hygiene day fully scheduled so you can go beyond your production goals. And your patients will be happy because you'll continue to treat them with "white-glove" service (Fig. 11.4).

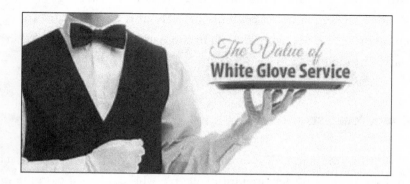

Figure 11.4 — The value of good service

A Hygienepreneur is a hygiene care manager, hygiene schedule manager, patient advocate, and the supreme practice builder. As a key producer in the practice, we hygienists are forced to study our schedules constantly to make sure they are full and productive. We have to be able to dodge and weave when schedules are full and not-so-full. When our schedules have gaps, there are tricks to fill those openings to keep the day productive.

We have all experienced times in dental hygiene work when schedules fall apart and we need help. Being ready to take action with the skills to maneuver and adjust during these moments is a pillar of excellence that a Hygienepreneur must strive to achieve. Being proactive with this and taking action is the first step in taking charge of your day and showing your doctor, and your patients, that you really care about them and the practice.

So, knowing that, how do you best "save" your schedule, one appointment at a time?

CHAPTER 12
"Saving" the Schedule, One Hygiene Appointment at a Time

So it's a Monday morning, and we've all been there: we walk in thinking that our schedule is completely full, just as it was on Friday when we left work, or on the Thursday before. But now patients are calling in with different reasons to cancel their appointments. As your front office is taking the calls and trying to facilitate filling those openings, a secondary plan of action can go into effect. You can help yourself by making a plan like that.

It's wonderful when opportunities occur that can enable you to provide service that you might not have had time to do for a patient who is in your schedule. Taking the initiative to engage in opportunities like that is the key to turning your day around, one appointment at a time.

It is important to spend the first fifteen minutes of your day reviewing your patients' history, and invaluable in being able to look for potential treatment needs and patient care opportunities. Sometimes we see a patient who needs extra services, such as limited scaling and root planing, or laser therapy to help reduce inflammation.

Let's face it: as dental hygienists, we're masters at doing a lot of procedures in a limited time period, though timing has always been a challenge for us! It is still our job as a clinical provider to promote exceptional quality of care during the time of service. But we also drive the success of our own schedules—the other team members are not going to know that a patient needs limited scaling and root planing, or that there are other services that the patient may need.

The assessment comes from us—we are the ones who examine the patient and present our assessment of the care that is needed to our doctors. It is very simple: if you have the time and they have a need, do the dentistry. You will get the "yes" from the patient if they are sitting in your chair. They have already taken the time to be there, so if you have extra time because your schedule has openings, then do the care that the patient needs right then—at that appointment, on that day (Fig. 12.1). The presentation to do the extra care for the patient is easy.

It could be said like this:

HYGIENIST: "Mr. Smith, I've just completed your assessment and it looks like these areas on the upper right and lower left are in need of extra therapy. Sometimes, areas are in need of extra care to promote healing. The procedure that is necessary is limited, and will promote healing, which is what we need. Inflammation in the gums is treated more proactively now that we can correlate this to inflammation in the body. We view oral health and your overall systemic health as one in the same. We want to prevent the further destruction of gum and bone, but we also want to prevent heart issues, diabetes and strokes.

The care is to follow through with what we are doing. We see you every three months for maintenance and you are using the proper tools to take care of yourself at home. However, sometimes, every few years we need to target specific areas with root smoothing when they are not healing, and we need to remove diseased tissue in those pockets to promote healing. We also disinfect these areas with laser therapy. After that, we will bring you back in six weeks to check the specific problem areas to make sure they are healthier and stable. Fortunately, I have the time today to do the care that these areas are needing to promote gum and bone health. It won't take me that much time, and we can get it all done for you and save you a visit back. How does that sound?"

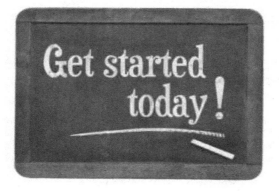

Figure 12.1 — Going ahead with work
when your schedule permits it

Chances are that when a patient is already in the chair, the "yes" will come easier. He or she is already seated and ready to go. Just grab the additional tools required and get to work. In the meantime, your front office will be working on filling any extra time availability that day by utilizing their short call lists. As providers, we will take the opportunity to deliver five-star service at an more relaxed pace, which reduces our stress level as well. Taking the opportunity to deliver extra care that the patient may need that day instead of rescheduling for another time is a win-win for everyone, and it's how we are practicing both as awesome Hygienepreneurs and as amazing care providers.

We are promoting the necessary care, all while helping our doctors' revenue, which helps our own income as well. After all, we not only became practicing clinicians to help others, but also to generate an equitable income for ourselves and our families. We want to be productive and at the same time be utilized to help others. When there are openings in the schedule, think of those as opportunities to take your care to the next level. The patient will think you are a superstar because you took care of everything they needed right then and there, and saved them another visit.

Making sure that all possible treatment needs for that patient are satisfied is how to "win" in your daily schedule. Again, if you have openings in your schedule and can start a root planing procedure, or complete adult sealants where necessary, or complete another adjunct that they may need—and you can complete it now that you have the time—then you should do it.

Another way to optimize an unexpectedly open schedule (Fig. 12.2) is when patients bring their child with them for their visit. If the child needs hygiene care, offer to take care of that as well. It will fill an opening in your schedule and it will accommodate the parent, who won't have to come back with the child on another day. To that parent, you will truly look like you are doing everything in your power to make it easier on them.

You can make it look easy and the flow can be expressed like this:

HYGIENIST: "Marilyn, this is so awesome. I just noticed that your son is in need of his hygiene appointment. If you would like...so you don't have to come back... I can take care of him after I see you. It won't take long and that will save you both a visit. We realize how busy you are!"

Your patient does not need to know that you had a hole in your schedule, or anything except that you are available for them, and that your aim is to deliver the optimum care for them. That typically makes a patient very happy and satisfied. Something that I learned when I was a waitress, long before my dental career, was that the front of the house should never know that there are problems in the back of the house: if there were problems in the kitchen, then the hostess and wait staff never allowed the customers to know about them. That should be a rule of thumb at a dental office too. This approach is meant to make the front-of-the-house experience for the patient the very best.

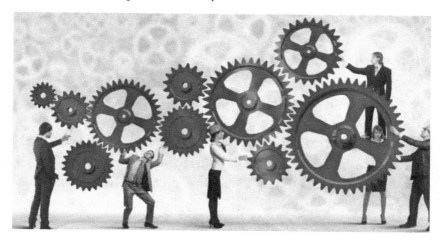

Figure 12.2 — Optimizing your schedule

I remember working at La Costa Resort and Spa when a guest requested a special kind of ice cream sandwich that was made back east—two delicious super chocolaty brownies filled with walnuts, with the best gourmet vanilla ice cream layered in between. Our guest was a celebrity tennis player who would have been displeased if I told her that we were out of the sandwich. But I took her order, knowing we were out, and smiled as I walked away, even though I was not sure where to get it. I just knew that it would be done!

We were trained never to say "no," or "I can't," to a guest. Their wishes were granted with a smile, every time. I had a plan that I was hoping would work, but had to follow through quickly: I knew of a high-end, gourmet grocery store that carried the desserts nearby. I told the chef I would be right back, then jumped on a golf cart and drove to the nearby plaza where the grocery store was located. Lo and behold, they had it! I drove back quickly, and had the chef sprinkle the top with some powdered sugar and place a few raspberries on the side. The guest was stoked! She had no idea what I had to do to get her the decadent dessert, and I didn't want her to know all the effort it took to deliver the five-star service. All she needed to know was that the service was given and presented with a smile. She returned every year and always ordered the same dessert.

In dentistry, our service should be delivered in the same exact spirit.

Our patients don't need to know that our schedules sometimes fall apart. They should assume that we are super booked and busy. We want them to have this idea in the back of their minds so that they are less likely to cancel their appointments, imagining they might get pushed out for months and become overdue. Similarly, our patients should never know about our supply problems, or lack of supplies. They should always feel confident that we have everything we need to take care of them in full.

The lesson of this chapter is basically to take control, take the time to manage your schedule, and look beyond what is already there. If you help your patient and help your practice, you'll help yourself in the end. There's nothing worse than a provider sitting around when they could be producing. Let's face it, our hands are highly skilled, and worth a lot of money, so when they're not in use it is very disappointing. We went to school for a long time, passing exams that were not easy; the time out in the field has prepared us for situations like these. We should be proactive, take control, and help our offices.

Another example of how we can help fill our own schedules is by thinking creatively and working with the patients who we have in our chairs (Fig. 12.).

I've often been doing a cleaning and have looked up from the patient to my computer and seen schedule changes happening for the afternoon. Then I think of the person in my chair right now: well, maybe her husband or children are due and need an appointment. I will ask her how that family member is doing and tell her that I would love to see them—I might even gently mention to her that I've had an unexpected change to my schedule, and if her family member wanted to come in today, I would love to see them.

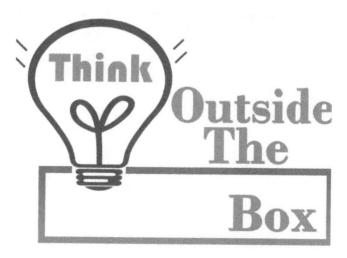

Figure 12.3 — Creative thinking to save a schedule

Sometimes I will even have that patient in the chair text their family member for me, expressing that there was an opening today and asking if they want to come in! It's amazing how many appointments I've filled on my own, just by talking to my patient who is in my chair at that moment.

My front office really appreciates it when a hygienist can help fill the schedule. Helping my team is a high-priority goal. Any way that I can take something off of their list of calls and follow-ups, and help them do other things to help our practice is a plus. A true Hygienepreneur thinks outside the box to promote the practice in any way possible, all while delivering great patient care!

Scheduling for yourself is important—we want our reappointment rate as close to 100% as possible, and to keep our schedules full. If a hygienist schedules from her operatory herself, the patient is more likely to keep the appointment, knowing that they have a reserved appointment with you. That personal touch ensures that they will show up because they want to see you, and they don't want to let you down.

That all leads us to scheduling *smart*. How do you best do that?

CHAPTER 13
Scheduling Smart: Not Just an Automatic Schedule

You know your schedule best, and you know how much time you need per patient type. Who is more difficult to treat? Who needs more care? Who likes to talk a lot? Who needs more procedures? You know all of this valuable information. This is why you need to be in charge of your schedule, not just be filling in one-size-fits-all schedule blocks that some system assigns.

As hygienists, we need to ask if we really need an hour for every patient. If we really think about it and we look at all the different types of patients we see and the different types of procedures that we do, let's be honest: do they all require an hour? I am a firm believer in looking at your own schedule and being realistic about how much time you need. We are often rushed in the jobs that we do, so we don't want to shortchange ourselves, or the patient. But there are some instances where a patient doesn't need an exam, or doesn't need X rays. Why? Because they take really good care of their teeth at home, with fantastic oral hygiene, and may have a low rate of caries (Fig. 13.1). We can realistically clean patients like that in 45 minutes without appearing rushed.

If we schedule in a way that is customized for each procedure and each patient, we can be more productive during the day. Fitting one or two extra patients into your daily schedule can turn a day from unproductive to productive. We should be open to this, and open to thinking outside of the box. As Hygienepreneurs, all of us need to find ways to keep ourselves productive in our practice. This is another reason to be in charge of your schedule and schedule your patients' next visit on your own. For example, if you are scheduling a child for his next hygiene appointment (Fig. 13.2), and you know that he is probably going to be needing sealants on his next visit, you can customize the amount of time needed during that appointment and plan on adding the sealants.

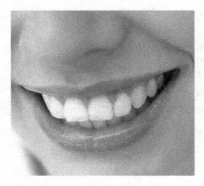

Figure 13.1 — Customize the appointment time based on need

Pre-scheduling certain procedures that you know a patient will need helps your time management because you can make sure that you have the supplies for it set up in advance. You can also make sure you have time scheduled for that procedure so that you can do it on that day, and not on another day. We have to pay attention to both our patients' current needs and future needs. Hygienepreneurs are always thinking about how to boost the patient's health and at the same time, boost the productivity of the appointment. As a hygienist, you are the only one who knows how much time that patient really needs. You may need less time for one patient, or you may need more time for another. When you schedule the patient's next visit, you can customize that based upon what you need and what that patient needs. If patients need an exam and X rays at their next visit, then you may want to schedule more time for that.

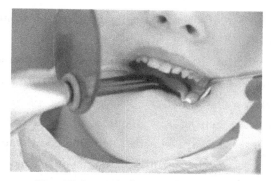

Fig. 13.2 — Working with children

Also, if you have a patient who is more difficult to take care of, you may need more time for that patient as well. Customizing your schedule based on need, and not just an automatic hour, is smart business. Not every hygienist takes charge of her schedule, but when they schedule their own patients, it will alleviate the unknown from the front office. All hygienists should regularly look at their schedules in advance to modify them and make changes that need to happen.

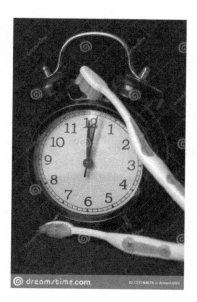

Figure 13.3 — Customizing your schedule

If a patient calls in and schedules an appointment, and you notice that the front office didn't allow for enough time, or scheduled too much time, then modify and customize the appointment. Time is extremely valuable, and every minute should be accounted for, just as it is for our doctors. It works amazingly well when we can have a meeting with our scheduling coordinator and let them know what our "soft parameters" are for each type of patient. I have worked with scheduling coordinators who will write these down for each hygienist because, again, each one practices a little differently. That way the coordinator can just follow the guidelines for each hygienist, and the hygienist can make it a normal routine to go through the schedule to make sure that all the patients are scheduled for the appropriate amount of time. Each day can be more productive when we can practice more efficiently. When patients get their needs met, the practice wins, and the hygienist looks amazing!

K. Pat Brown, DDS puts it this way: "Understanding that your hourly production goal should be three times your hourly wage changes how you look at scheduling."

CHAPTER 14
Dissecting Your Appointment Time to Stay on Schedule and Complete All Tasks

As hygienists, we live and die by time increments—we fear making our patients wait for their appointments, and we strive to be five minutes ahead of schedule in order to train our patients to be on time as well. If we are constantly late for them, we risk patients remembering this and showing up late for us on their next visits because they think we won't be on time. This is a "global" hygiene issue that's the number one topic of discussion in the field. But, there is a saving grace. We can follow definite systems to almost eliminate this issue from creeping up in our offices.

Most practices operate on a one hour schedule. So the hygienists need to sit down with their doctors and determine what needs to happen within that hour, down to the minute. How long does it take to set up and break down your room? How long does it take to perform the greeting process, updated health questions, and complete the X rays, intraoral images, and periodontal assessment? How long do you need to scale and polish? Lastly, how long does your doctor need to complete his exam? All of these procedures need to be analyzed.

We need to be realistic about how much time we actually need, and stay focused on the goal of getting things done according to the schedule. Of course, there are going to be exceptions to the rule, but if we follow guidelines that have been planned by the entire practice, then we will stay on time (Fig. 14.1).

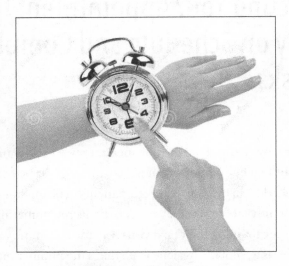

Figure 14.1 — Staying on time

So, with all of that taken care of, then you need to make sure that the procedure that you're doing for your patients is the proper one. If you find you need more time on a patient because the pocket probing depths are extensive, with bleeding and a huge amount of debris, then that patient needs to be reassessed for a different procedure that allows for more time. And you'll need to bill for it!

Assessing patients properly not only provides great quality of care for their overall health, but also helps keep the schedule healthy. Experts know that in an adult-based practice, the ratio should be 70% perio to 30% prophy on average—meaning that 70% of your adult patients will be involved periodontally. When we determine the proper care for them, we are not only protecting their oral health but also protecting the health of their overall body.

Over and over again it has been reported that periodontal disease links to many other medical issues (Fig. 14.2). It puts the patient at a higher risk for comorbidities such as diabetes and heart disease, along with many other systemic diseases. For that reason it should not be left untreated, or swept underneath the rug. In fact, most hygienists and doctors are now more aggressive than ever when it comes to the treatment of this terrible disease. That's another reason why it is inappropriate to switch back and forth between perio and prophy procedures.

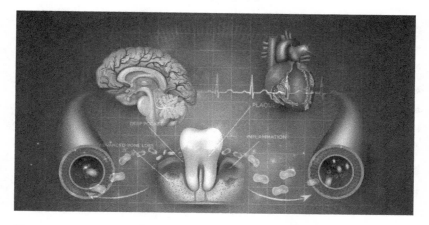

Figure 14.2 — The effects of periodontal disease on systemic health

First, we need to classify patients properly. Once a patient is classified as perio, he or she is always perio. Not only do we need to categorize our patients properly, but we must also plan for and allow the necessary time to deliver the necessary care (Fig. 14.3). When we find that we are scaling prophy patients time and time again because the case is more difficult than expected, then the team needs to revisit and modify the office perio guidelines. This modification will result in accurate coding, better time management, and enhanced quality of care.

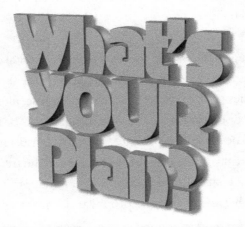

Figure 14.3 — The importance of classifying and planning

Second, most hygienists that I interview say that their problems with staying on time develop when their doctor doesn't come in right away for the exam, or talks too much during their exam. Patients due for an exam sometimes have to wait for the doctor to come in and do his thing. As hygienists, we feel so bad when the doctor is running between a couple of his own rooms, and we don't want him to feel pressured—we know what that feels like.

The best way to handle incorporating the recare exam into a hygiene appointment is for the Hygienepreneur to finish X rays and a complete assessment at the very start of the appointment. The doctor should then come in whenever it is convenient for him. If we wait until the hygiene appointment is almost finished for the doctor to come in, the hygienist usually ends up running late.

So, as a hygienist, ask for the patient exam whenever it's convenient for the doctor. It may work better to have the doctor do the exam in the first ten minutes of the appointment, or in the final ten minutes. You and your doctor should communicate this plan with each other before patients arrive.

Being prepared for your doctors to come in whenever they can break away, whether you are finished working or not, is an advantage. Discussing the proposed plan for the day in the morning huddle is key. It's a great time to identify patients who need encouragement from the doctor to accept treatment recommendations. Letting your doctors know what they can expect when they walk in will allow for better time management, a more thorough exam, and better communication for everyone.

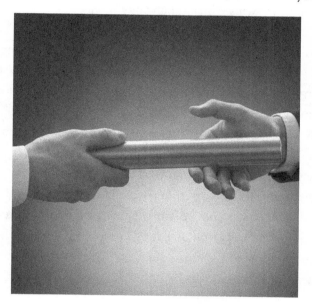

Fig. 14.4 — Working with your doctor to develop an efficient handoff

Decide in advance how much time your doctor needs for an exam to make sure he is staying on track. Your handoff to him should be short, organized, practiced, and synchronized to the time allotted for the exam (Fig. 14.4). When you are delivering your initial handoff to the doctor, encourage him to just listen. Time management together improves when you are not interrupting each other and backtracking. Have all the records, X rays, and charts up and ready for him so the transition is smooth. Stay on task, follow the system, and your timing will be precise.

If something happens, and your doctor still has not come in, quietly put a little note up in his room signaling that you are ready. If that doesn't work, ask the assistant if you can move your patient into another room for the exam. Anticipating both of your schedules is key to running on time. Knowing what's going on with his schedule will help you anticipate snags. If you see potential issues coming up, you can act accordingly and shift the current system to another system so that everybody's needs are met and everyone wins—including your patients.

In a scenario like the one above, be calm, smile, and ask the patient to follow you down to the other room where the doctor can see them. (Don't forget to schedule your patient's next appointment before leaving your room!) Once the patient is seated in the other room, hand off all information to your assistant. This will promote good communication practices with the doctor because the assistant will then do the handoff, explaining everything you saw and did for the patient. Before you leave patients with your teammates, though, let them know you look forward to seeing them the next time, reassure them that they are in great hands, then exit. Now you will be on time for your next patient, which reduces your stress and helps you start your next patient's appointment in a positive way and on time, which in itself is a practice builder.

Remember that you are a Hygienepreneur, someone who is managing a schedule well. You're flexible when situations occur beyond your control, and you adjust to those changes with ease when necessary. Customizing appointment times for each patient and each appointment type is a huge plus when trying to meet your goal of practicing smarter and not harder and winning every day.

Now, let's discuss hygiene scheduling with a purpose!

CHAPTER 15
Hygiene Scheduling with a Purpose: Why the Hour Time Slot Is So Passé

Long ago, when I worked in the front office at a dental practice, every hygiene appointment was one hour long. If it was a scaling and root planning appointment, it was ninety minutes for just half of the patient's mouth. All children were scheduled for thirty minutes. It was like clockwork. But those days of automatic scheduling everyone in a "cookie cutter" slot are long over. Scheduling is now customized by procedure, and also by patient.

As you probably know, a prophy on a twenty-one-year old is usually easier to do than the same procedure on patients in their late sixties with multiple restorations. When we are older, we may have areas that take longer to clean due to existing crowns and bridges. Patients who are older may need periomaintenance therapy cleaning if they have areas of recession, bone loss, and concavities that take longer to adapt to and scale smoothly. Some elderly patients may be medically compromised, and have tartar buildup, stain, and interproximal food traps that require more time to clean.

"As a dentist, I have learned to schedule time needed not based on procedure code," says K. Pat Brown, DDS. "Hygiene should do the same."

For example, scheduling an hour-long prophylaxis for a twenty-one-year old with no exam and no X rays is sometimes not necessary. As a hygienist, you know your patients. If you schedule according to procedure and need (Fig. 15.1), you will have a more productive day and deliver higher quality care with less stress.

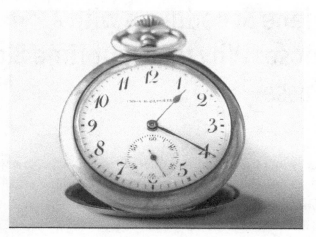

Figure 15.1 — Scheduling the time that's appropriate

If you need more time, schedule it, but if you need less time, then by all means, schedule for that. The standard "eight-patient day" will increase to ten, but that extra two patients can transform a day, moving it into the territory of surpassing your daily goal.

As a Hygienepreneur, you're doing great quality care while working more efficiently and turning a profit for the practice. It is important for all hygienists to manage their schedules and make sure those schedules always surpass the daily productivity goal.

Not all practices have bonus systems set up for their hygienists. I encourage bonus systems for all providers (Fig. 15.2). The standard hourly goal is usually calculated as the hourly salary of the hygienist times three. So, if a hygienist's hourly wage is $40 per hour, then the production goal would be $120. The practice would offer a predetermined percentage of anything over goal. If you produce $150 for the hour, then you would earn a percentage of the additional $30. More offices calculate all of the hours in the pay period and figure out what the goal is; anything over that, which the hygienist produces, would earn them some percentage on top of their hourly wage. This incentive is very motivating. When the schedule is full and productive, the office and hygienist are equally happy because they both win!

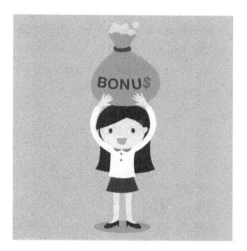

Figure 15.2 — Bonus: a little extra on top

If your office adopts a bonus system on top of your hygiene salary, you'll see an increase in the hygiene department revenue. People naturally work harder and more efficiently and are willing to say yes to doing extra work when they have a vested interest in the results.

Note to Doctors—Embrace your hygiene team! Support your team as they become Hygienepreneurs. Your practice and patients will win every time. I have always urged hygienists to control their own schedules. Every patient who leaves your office needs to leave with a hygiene appointment too. As care providers, your hygienists know what is involved with each patient and how much time that patient needs for them for the next visit, so encourage them to schedule it.

As providers, when we schedule patients for their next visit, it makes their commitment to show up at their next visit more personal. Your "no show" rate will be reduced because patients won't want to back out of the commitment that they made with their favorite hygienist. A Hygienepreneur not only does this, but also schedules patients back for their next visit and continues to deliver the best quality care with the offering of adjunct procedures. The hygiene department should be run as its own entity within the practice—a "practice within the practice." A hygiene-driven practice promotes less stress on the doctor. So as a hygienist, manage your practice and you will see the fruits of your labor (Fig. 15.3)!

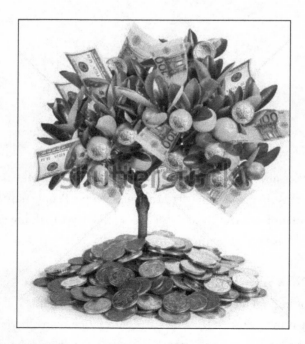

Figure 15.3 — Good scheduling will bear fruit

Managing Your Schedule and Taking Control of Your Income

Adjunct procedures are procedures such as fluoride treatment, whitening impressions, nightguard impressions, laser therapy and the placement of antibiotic therapy. Adult and child sealant placement is an awesome procedure that can reduce the need for more advanced procedures. Adjuncts add up in a big way after you evaluate your day (Fig. 15.4). There are several ways to manage your schedule the way you want to:

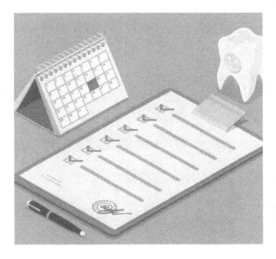

Figure 15.4 — Checklist for adjunct procedures

First, reappoint all your patients for their next hygiene appointments the day you see them.

- Second, go through your existing schedules and make sure X rays, fluoride and antibiotic therapy and laser therapy are added where necessary.
- Third, check to see if your perio maintenance therapy patients are in need of limited or full quadrants of SRP.
- Fourth, if a night guard was recommended by your doctor, anticipate taking the necessary impressions that day..

- Finally, ask the patient if they are ready to have their trays made and a full whitening kit delivered.

Remind them that the best time to whiten their teeth is after a cleaning and thorough polish. If they say "yes" then that will boost your hourly production as well.

Taking control of your schedule is the way to be a true Hygienepreneur. Success will follow and a more fulfilling career will be evident. It all starts with your schedule. Manage it and your days of practice will be less stressful and more rewarding.

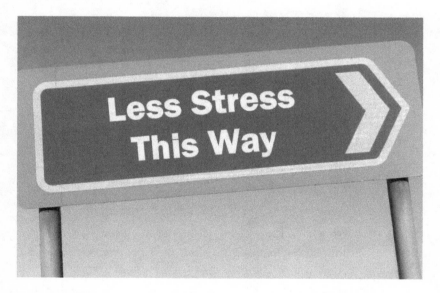

Figure 15.5 — Schedule your way to a less stressful day

It only takes a few minutes to schedule your patient's next hygiene visit. Don't ask her if you can schedule it, tell her with confidence, "Okay, Mrs. Jones, let's go ahead and reserve your next hygiene appointment so that you get the time that is convenient for you." If the patient says, "No, I don't know my schedule," respond "That's okay, let's set up a tentative time for you to come back. It's part of the recall system that we have here in the office. If we need to change it when it gets closer that will be okay."

Your reappoint rate should be 100% unless the patient you are seeing is leaving the practice due to a move. Even college student patients can be scheduled. Take the time to look up their college calendars and propose a date and time. No patient should leave your chair without an appointment.

Gary Kadi, *author of Million Dollar Dentistry*, recommends that you

> *aim for 100 percent pre-appointments before your patients leave. Get them back into the computer immediately – don't let them out of the system. This is another "bleeding point" in the practice. Make sure that everybody gets a card one month before an appointment, a call two weeks before and then a call forty-eight hours in advance of the appointment. If you've got people who say, "I don't know what my schedule is going to be," simply be proactive with them.*

It's all in the phrasing you use. Saying, "Let's go ahead and make your next appointment" instead of asking them permission to do so, will ensure that you will get the "yes." Your schedule for the day should be set up for success.

Remember that you are the Hygienepreneur. You are in charge of your own schedule and your high production destiny. Going through your schedule one week in advance, and then the day before, and double-checking it the morning of the appointment as well will ensure that all the procedures that you can do in their appointment time will be completed. Making sure that X rays, adult fluoride, sealants on kids and adults (if previously recommended), laser therapy for perio involved patients, and the correct procedure codes are entered are keys to high productivity.

Make sure that any periapicals are noted as well. If you are doing a checkup on images of four bitewings and three PA's (Fig. 15.6), then make sure that all the images you enter can be billed.

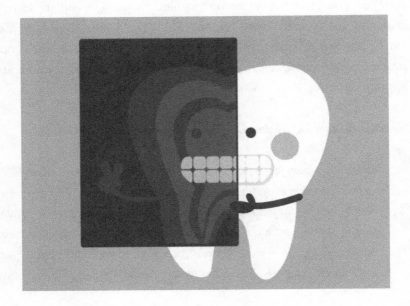

Figure 15.6 — Auditing periomaintenance

Your front office will appreciate the help with this quick audit, and your daily production will increase with just a few clicks of the mouse. This holds true for your periomaintenance therapy patients who have not had scaling and root planing done in a while. Some insurance companies now require SRP to be done every two to three years to continue to establish a periodontal need. Ask your front office to check in advance the frequency limitations for this procedure, and treat areas as necessary, following up with laser therapy. Even if the roots are rough in a limited amount of teeth, present a treatment plan and complete the work.

Knowing in advance when your perio patients are due or eligible will aid in time management. You can anticipate the need and treat the areas where necessary, saving your patient a visit back and streamlining the financial arrangement process as well—which also helps with time management. We are always pressed for time, so by pre-prepping your day and looking over your schedule for possible needs, you will be surprised with the extra care you are able to deliver, all while maintaining a steady schedule.

I am not saying that you should allow the insurance company to dictate the dental plan. Whether a procedure is covered or not should not affect your assessment or treatment. The patient's needs come first. What I am suggesting is that you use your pre-knowledge of what's covered and not covered to make a quick decision, and treat the areas that need to be treated in a timely manner, with efficiency. Plan ahead, so that financial arrangements can be made quickly that allow you to get the "yes" and move forward with the care that you would like to deliver.

Now, on to Part IV, which covers how to use adjunct procedures to increase patient health and practice growth!

IV. ADJUNCTS FOR INCREASING PATIENT HEALTH & PRACTICE GROWTH

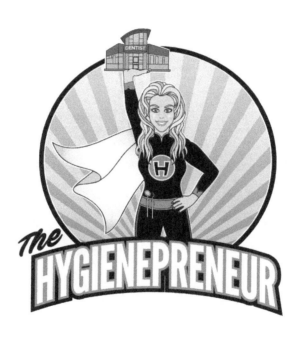

CHAPTER 16
Adjunct Procedures that Boost Your Level of Care and Profitability

Adjunct procedures are huge when it comes to meeting your goals of increasing your daily production. When a tooth is treated with a sealant, filling the deep pits in with material can help prevent tooth decay. Adult sealants are generally not a covered benefit by most insurance companies, but preventing the loss of tooth structure (and thereby reducing the patient's time in the chair and money spent) is enough reason to continue to prevent, prevent, prevent. After all, we eat right and exercise to prevent physical ailments, so why wouldn't we promote prevention procedures for our teeth as well?

With your doctor, come up with a plan of action for your patients. If adult sealants are not covered, decide on a fee in advance so you are ready to quickly present it and treat the tooth as necessary. Adult sealants are so easy to do—you are treating an adult, not a child, and the procedure is completed very easily. It is a wonderful service that you are giving to your patients. They will appreciate you, and your practice will see financial benefits as well.

K. Pat Brown, DDS says it is important to begin "switching the paradigm from pocket reduction only to a more comprehensive oral health plan including inflammation reduction and root decay prevention, [which] requires multiple adjunct hygiene procedures."

If a patient presents a financial issue, simply come up with a fee that is reasonable and offer it. Be sure to stress that preventing a filling in the future is very beneficial, and suggest that you "can have it done today to save them an appointment," which is always a courteous and effective way to communicate it. Remember, it's all about customer service and convenience. You will get the "yes" if you make it easy on the patient.

Performing adjunct procedures helps practitioners in our field operate above the standard of care. It is important for us to practice the way we want to practice, but we should always be mindful of the challenges that insurance companies present on a daily basis. As a guiding industry philosophy, we should not allow them to dictate what we offer and don't offer. Remember, they are trying to increase their profits, and aren't really looking out for patients, regardless of what they say. We want to allow our patients to decide and choose the level of dental health care they sign up for. The patient is in charge! We are just there to guide and inform.

You should evaluate possible preventive procedures for every patient on your schedule so that you are doing the most that you can for them in the time that you have. Consider the following seven adjunct procedures for every patient:

1. Adult fluoride treatment. In-office Adult fluoride treatments (Fig. 16.1) are great for the patient who suffers from sensitivity, has root exposure, and has crowns, bridges and fillings that need to be maintained. A patient with a high rate of caries, or decalcification, should also be considered for this preventive procedure. Tell the patient that fluoride is "not just for kids" anymore. The ADA and doctors everywhere are recommending this procedure now more than ever to protect and prevent tooth decay.

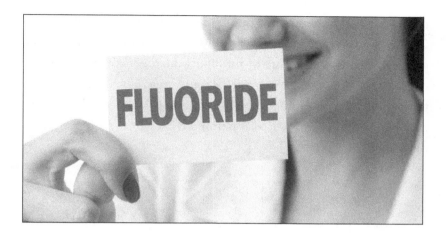

Figure 16.1 — Adult fluoride treatment as an adjunct procedure

2. *Bonded desensitizer treatment.* Two available products that are recommended are Seal and Protect, by Dentsply, and Brush and Bond, by Parkell. Both products are equally useful and effective and have a fluoride releasing action that works very well. If your patient has a root sensitive area (Fig. 16.2) that shows up after their dental cleaning, this

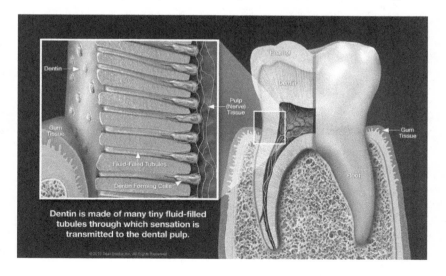

Figure 16.2 — Tooth sensitivity

procedure can be completed on that tooth or teeth, and a fee can be assessed for this procedure. (You would use code D9910, "Application of desensitizing medicament," for billing purposes). If the insurance company does not cover it, come up with a fee that is reasonable for the patient and your practice. This adjunct procedure will help the patient clinically, and will also help increase your billing per hour, per patient.

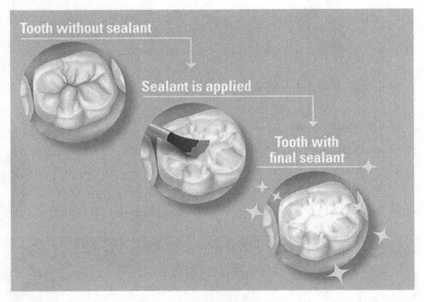

Figure 16.3 — Applying tooth sealants

3. Adult sealants. Placing a sealant is an easy way to protect a tooth with deep grooves. This procedure is recommended for patients who have a high occlusal caries rate and who have deep pits in their teeth. It can quickly be done during a routine hygiene appointment and easily performed by the hygienist. It can sometimes be challenging to place sealants on children, but adult patients typically cooperate, opening their mouths nice and wide, and the treatment literally takes less than five minutes to complete.

Think about it: hygienists have placed sealants on children for years. Why can't we do it for adults as well? We should. The difference is you sometimes need to treat the adult tooth first with a prophy jet. The high pressured water and baking soda polishes out extrinsic stains that might be present, and prepares the tooth for the sealant. Of course, it is important to check the patient's insurance to see the frequency for placement and replacement allowed, but that shouldn't be a roadblock for treatment.

Placing sealants on permanent first and second molars is so important (Fig. 16.3). With children, preventing tooth decay in those early stages when their dexterity is challenged is a plus. In the past, if we placed a sealant on a tooth once, we would never look at it again to reseal it if a pit was exposed or the retention was compromised.

As a provider, it is important to be proactive in setting up your day for success. Check with your insurance coordinator to review patient history for sealants and replacement frequency; it is much better to know the benefits available for the procedure before the patient arrives in order to manage your time better so you actually have time to do the procedure. Time is money, as Ben Franklin said, and if we have to wait for insurance verification, we may not have time to complete the care that is recommended. So anticipate what care may be needed, know the patients' coverage for it, and be ready to communicate it when they come in for their visit. Anticipation and preparation increases patient care and productivity!

4. Laser periodontal treatments. Lasers can be used to help reduce inflammation and fight gum disease. This procedure is extremely important for patients' periodontal stability and prevention of future periodontal surgery.

"For you, the dental hygienist," Mike Czubiak, DDS and Steve Sperry write, "the two most common uses of the diode laser (Fig. 16.4) are to reduce the bacterial load in the pockets during a maintenance appointment and to remove diseased tissue, granulation tissue, in the pockets during scaling and root planing (SRP) appointments."

Laser bacterial reduction aids in the reduction of bacteria colonies and helps tighten the tissue, creating a seal around the root. When the mode of the laser is changed to the *Degranulation of Diseased Tissue* setting, diseased tissue can be removed with ease using an activated tip. The laser gently and effectively cuts diseased, pigmented tissue from within the periodontal pocket. The results can be amazing. The tissue should form a seal around the root, creating a shallower pocket. This treatment also reduces inflammation. Preventing further destruction of bone and gum is key to preventing additional problems in the future. Remember, some patients are very fearful of having to see a periodontist. They will be eager to prevent surgery, if possible. When the laser is presented as a preventative measure, you should get the "yes."

K. Pat Brown, DDS says, "The *yes* does not need to come in the first contact with the patient. When presenting adjuncts, some patients need to hear it more than once. Document and point out issues that can be improved, and when they do say yes, they will be committed."

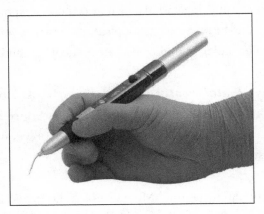

Figure 16.4 — Dental diode laser

5. *Antibiotic treatments.* Another adjunct procedure that helps prevent periodontal disease is the placement of antibiotics under the gum line where tissue is red and not healing, especially after scaling and root planing is completed.

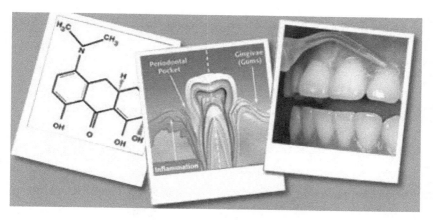

Figure 16.5 — Antibiotic treatments

Antibiotic therapies, such as Arestin, are a fantastic adjunct procedure and can be done every three months to help maintain gum and bone health (Fig 16.5). Arestin is placed under the gum line in a pre-dosed capsule of minocycline HCL 1mg microspheres. When the powder mixes with the moisture in the pocket, it turns into a solid. The antibiotic is then able to work in a time-released state, administering antibiotic over a ten-day period, which helps the gum in the area get healthier.

Mike Czubiak, DDS and Steve Sperry offers this overview:

There have been several locally applied subgingival antimicrobials that have made their way to the market. A resorbable gelatin matrix containing chlorhexidine gluconate called PerioChip has been around for a while with some good results. It releases CHX for 7-10 days and has been shown to improve pocket depths and bleeding over nine months. Subgingival doxycycline (Atridox) and subgingival minocycline (Arestin) have seen similar positive results including reduction of bleeding points, increase in clinical attachment level and probing depths. These subgingival antimicrobials should always be used as adjuncts to scaling and root planing. This will ensure that there will be a reduction in bacteria as well as in the body's inflammatory response.

As with laser treatments, the hygienist should be realistic with the patient as to whether or not this procedure will need to be done every three months to ensure proper periodontal health.

Regardless of whether a hygiene procedure is covered by the insurance company, it should always be offered to the patient. Allowing the patient to decide is key. If the patient is in need of a fluoride treatment every time they come in, then tell them that. It is much easier to present it once than to have to keep offering it every three months. It is much easier to let them know that every three months they will need a procedure and that the fee is "x" amount of dollars per visit.

Saying it once instead of every time is way more efficient and will make our jobs easier. We are professionals who know how to treat our patients and know what our patients' needs are. So why not just share the message one time and make it easy on them? If we deliver this message once, and the patient accepts it, that will give us the time to discuss other things, dental related or not. Our time with them is valuable, and we need to be smart with this. So, share the information, move on, and gain a patient for life.

When you make the next appointment, document that the patient accepted the procedure to be done and the fee that is associated with the procedure. This is a great way to remind yourself that the patient has been informed, is aware of everything, and has bought into the plan. It's also a great way to let your front office staff know that the procedure and fee have been discussed and accepted (Fig. 16.6).

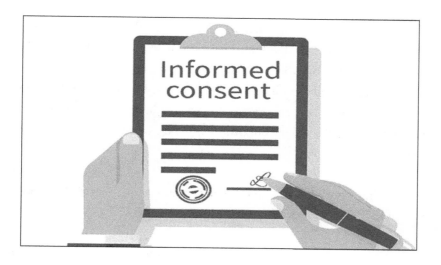

Figure 16.6 — Getting consent in advance for repeated treatments

6. *Whitening treatments.* Traditional whitening with take home trays, or in-office whitening with a product like Zoom, is also a great way to enhance patient happiness and your production with adjuncts. Take the initiative to suggest this and watch how many of your patients say yes. Whether they want to do it with you today or in the near future, it will benefit everyone. Taking impressions for whitening trays or the pre-procedural Zoom preparation trays only takes a few minutes. Your day will go from productive to super-productive, in the way that an associate dentist contributes to a practice. Those kinds of numbers are totally attainable. Suggest great care, save your patient an extra appointment, and win!

7. *Night guards.* Sometimes, when all of the patient's restorative care has been finished, he or she still needs a night guard that the dentist previously recommended. Finding out about the patient's insurance coverage for the appliance in advance, while preparing your day, is huge. If you know the fee, you can remind the patient that they need this, and can take the impression that day. Save your patient a visit back, enhance their care, and increase your production in less than fifteen minutes. Boom!

We have to be active and efficient. Our office will win when we help to protect the patients' teeth and existing dentistry from bruxism. As Hygienepreneurs, we must take action as a patient liaison, especially when we are dealing with PPO fee schedules. By delivering five-star patient care and winning every day (because adjuncts improve the health of our patients), we will see our production numbers grow and continue to practice excellence.

So, moving right along . . . let's next discuss how to deal with the fee schedules PPOs allow for hygiene procedures.

CHAPTER 17
The Numbers Game: How to Deal with PPO Hygiene Fee Schedules

Dealing with insurance is a huge topic at all dental conferences and lectures: Our doctors struggle to meet their goals and pay their bills because PPO fee schedules continue to be too low to pay for the care we need to offer patients in our practices (Fig. 17.1). It seems crazy that PPO fee schedules are still paying so little, but there are things we can do to ensure survival. Offering adjuncts (Chapter 16), along with proper hygiene assessment and diagnosis, correct billing and coding, careful time management, and keeping full schedules are all ways to combat this.

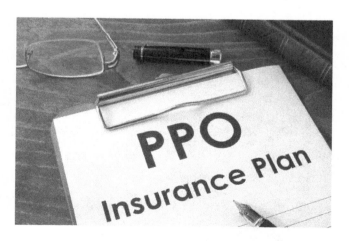

Figure 17.1 — Dealing with PPO limitations

"Unfortunately, insurance fees are being driven down," notes K. Pat Brown, DDS:

> *The hourly billing for a hairdresser can be higher than for a hygienist sometimes. To survive, we have to offer the best treatment and charge a fair fee outside of the insurance confines. At "usual and customary" rates, which is the doctor's highest fee level, a patient can have complementary services given to them. But at the PPO "discounted fee" schedule, there is no room for courtesies.*

We need to first make sure that we are billing and using the proper codes for what we do (Fig 17.2). Also, we need to encourage doctors to effectively negotiate with the insurance companies to make sure that our fees are updated and accurate. There is usually one person in the front office who keeps track of that process. They know when they last saw fees increased, which plans were affected, and when it will be time to do it again. You need to study each PPO fee schedule. As a professional, you must offer the best solutions and become comfortable with quoting fees.

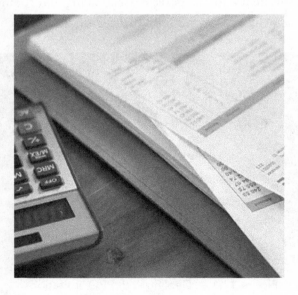

Figure 17.2 — Proper coding

Proper coding of procedures is important and helpful in learning how to effectively manage PPOs. Did you know that most doctors don't bill for everything that they do? It's true. This holds true for billing for personal protective equipment, even though dental offices have always operated at a higher standard of care using such equipment. Encourage your doctors to seek outside professional training on proper coding.

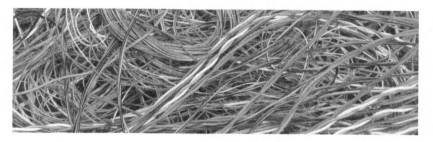

Figure 17.3 — Untangling the confusion of coding

When we focus on the specifics of what we do, and dissect each appointment down to the nitty gritty, we can take advantage of every opportunity to deliver great care—and bill for it (Fig. 17.3). It is imperative to look at the hygiene department as a winning, self-operating machine. Hygiene should be the foundation for the rest of the practice to build upon. The department can actually carry the rest of the practice and provide the constant residual income that can be counted upon. The hygiene machine also provides doctors the satisfaction of delivering great care to their patients as the patients' hygiene and restorative needs are fulfilled.

A stable hygiene department grows when it follows a systematic approach to patient care. Let it take on the lion's share of the work so the doctor can practice with ease, and under less pressure. With more hygienists, it will become necessary to add more doctors to support the practice. Your hygienists' production will help pay for that associate. Help drive that, and you will be a superstar in your doctor's eyes.

Now on to Section V, and mastery of the skills that can make the difference between being an ordinary hygienist and a true Hygienepreneur!

V. MASTERY: BECOMING A HYGIENEPRENEUR

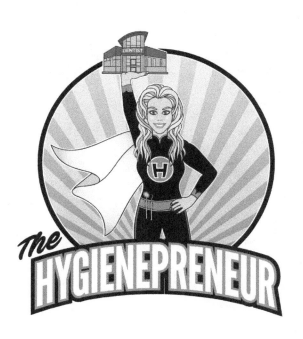

CHAPTER 18
Two Doctors & Three Hygienists: The Hierarchy

(Hint: In a Hygiene-Driven Practice, the Third Hygienist Pays for the Associate Dentist)

A common question and barrier to practice growth is, "When can I hire an associate doctor?" What I have found is that a well-trained third hygienist can pay their salary and the associate's salary, assuming you already have the available chair. Build the third hygienist's schedule first and add doctor days to match.
—K. Pat Brown, DDS

In the past, the dental hygiene department was a revenue-losing part of many practices. Doctors were happy if the hygiene schedules were full, regardless of what was actually being produced. Most days, the production that the hygienists were generating did not even cover their salaries. Its benefit was that the patient's periodontal health was being maintained and supported, but the revenue was in what was diagnosed for the doctor's schedule—fillings, crowns, bridges, and the like. Through recall exams, the doctor's schedule could be kept steady and busy.

Well, the days of the "Prophy Palace" are over! Times are very different in dentistry.

Insurance companies have made it much harder to succeed (Fig. 18.1). Insurance fee schedules have not kept up with inflation, dental supply costs, and salaries. The cost to run a dental practice has increased, while insurance companies are determined to pay less and less.

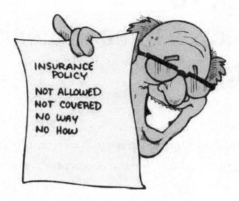

Figure 18.1 — Compensation from Dental Insurance Companies

Fortunately, most dentists have become savvy to this and are extremely passionate about "winning the battle." Here's where a Hygienepreneur comes in. A dentist's "time utilization" factor is extremely important. If he has a hygienist producing while he is doing other procedures, this is a very effective use of time. That's why tracking production is so important, and making sure that we are treating patients thoroughly and accurately is key.

Approximately 35% of codes billed to insurance companies from the hygiene department should be periodontal codes. In a practice, with an average mix of adults and children, the incidence of perio is about 40%—some say that this number can be as high as 60%. If 66% of your patients are adults, and 60% of them have periodontal involvement, then that number equates to about 39% of billing codes. So monitor this! If you find that number dropping, then a recalibration within your hygiene department will be necessary.

Revisiting the assessment process is always good. Make sure everyone is onboard and riding the horse the same way, which will help you manage and maintain your numbers. It will also keep those perio codes consistent if we are growing our new patient base in the practice. So, as hygienists, we need to watch our new patient numbers and keep track of the "back door" exits (patients who leave and never come back), which equals attrition.

We hygienists are a dynamic and hard-working bunch! We are helping our doctors win the insurance war and turn a profit, all while delivering great care. The time is now (Fig. 18.2).

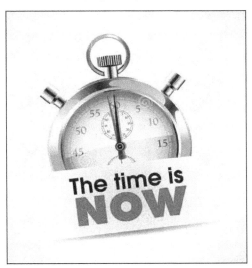

Figure 18.2 — Keeping up with your numbers

As hygienists, we need to pay attention to what we are doing for our patients and practice every day. Having this awareness is the first step. Looking at our schedules by the day, week, and month—although they are always changing—is important too. We should be leading the efforts to offset the limitations of insurance companies' fee schedules. Paying attention to our time allotments and procedures within the time allotments will help us work efficiently.

Just as our doctors track minute-by-minute time allotments per procedure, we need to do the same. How many minutes does it take to break down and set up a room? How many minutes does it take to greet the patient and take X rays? Each step in hygiene should be timed and managed. And, concurrent with that, each procedure that is done for each patient should be accounted for and billed accurately. The production goal for a hygienist should be to produce three times their hourly salary.

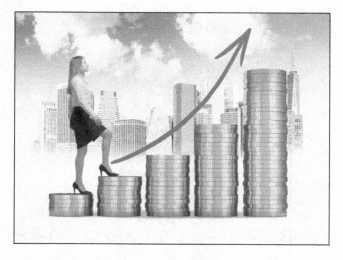

Figure 18.3 — Increasing production goals

By paying attention to what each patient needs, and ensuring that all procedures are entered and posted correctly, you will see success every day.

Doctors should be producing at least two times what the hygiene department is producing—when one hygienist is consistently producing $2,000 per day and the doctor is producing $4,000 per day, it's a great feeling! Can you imagine if your practice had two hygienists producing $2,000 every day? If that is done consistently, the third hygienist's production will pay for an associate dentist's salary. So, now the practice can have two doctors and three hygienists in place and be humming very efficiently.

Remember, approximately 60% to 75% of all restorative dental diagnoses are discovered during hygiene appointments. Hygienists are valuable on both the front end and the back end of the practice. We need to continue this process, "winning" for the practice and ourselves every day.

As K. Pat Brown, DDS noted at the beginning of this chapter, the common question about when it becomes possible to hire an associate doctor can often be answered by bringing in a well-trained third hygienist, who will pay for both her own salary and the associate's salary. After building the third hygienist's schedule, add doctor days to match.

Some hygienists have partnered up with dentists and work on an hourly rate, getting a bonus if certain production goals are hit. Production goals like these need to be reached in order for the practice to soar. When the hygienist hits her marks and makes extra money for the practice, she can put a portion of that into a bonus incentive plan. As a Hygienepreneur, you need to work to make that a reality for yourself, so be proactive and ask if an incentive program can be added to the practice. Although it's just a fraction of your total compensation, over time this adds up to become a huge benefit.

Become a Hygienepreneur and get a piece of the pie! It will create a sense of ownership and accountability that you will love. Everyone benefits from this, too. You practice with integrity for your patients and you work hard, so you should be paid for it in a way that makes you operate as if you own your department. That "ownership mentality" will make your doctor very happy when he sees the hygiene department's numbers at the end of the month, and sees that the patients are being treated so thoroughly. Help your patients and doctors and you will help yourself too!

So, now . . . how do you build a great dental hygiene team?

CHAPTER 19
Building a Great Dental Hygiene Team

Being surrounded by great teammates promotes a winning environment. If your environment is supportive, your goals will be met and your ability to practice will come easily. The goal is not just to practice smarter so that you soar financially, but also to practice with less stress, so your mental game is on point. We all want to operate at a reduced stress level. The mark of excellence is when hygienists reach their personal bests emotionally *and* financially. So, help build a team around you that will support you, with personalities that complement each other.

So, how do you do that?

I decided to write a chapter on hiring as one of the final pillars of attainment as a Hygienepreneur. If you want to become a lead hygienist and build a team of successful hygienists to surround you, you may be able to negotiate a higher salary to train and manage them. Encourage your doctor to carefully match teammates, so everyone's work environment is happy, fun and nurturing.

First, start with hiring the right team members—people with personality traits that gel with the existing team. Never just look at a résumé and do a perfunctory interview. An employee's experience and skill does make a huge difference, of course, but being selective about personality types is also very important if you want to keep your work life as calm and stress-free as possible. I have been very lucky to work with great doctors who had a gift for looking and working "outside of the box." I benefited from that in many ways. Several of these doctors, when they hired me or others, used different personality tests to determine how we'd fit in the practice.

Personality is so important! If an office has too many dominant "directors" and not enough "influencers" who are lively and motivating, then there could be conflict. I am sure that you have heard the saying, "too many cooks spoil the soup" (Fig. 19.1) Well, the same premise applies when developing a good team.

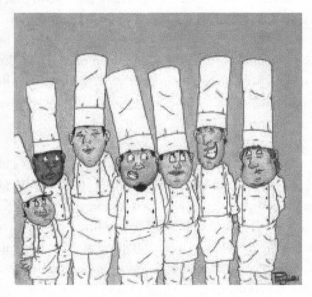

Figure 19.1 — Too many cooks?

Two personality evaluations that are very popular and used amongst many Fortune 500 companies are the DISC and Myers-Briggs tests.

The DISC (Dominance, Influence, Steadiness, Conscientiousness) system was created to help large and small companies enhance their executives' leadership and growth. It is often used for hiring, training, conflict manageability, guest services, and team bonding.

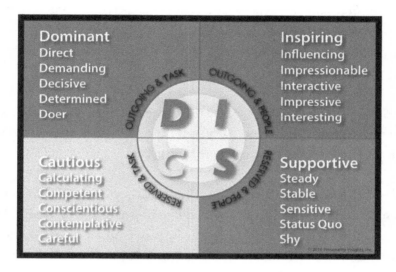

Figure 19.2 — The DISC matrix

The DISC test contains 28 questions. When I took it, for each question I was given a choice of words and asked to pick the one that was most like me. It was fast and easy. We took it as a team, and it was a lot of fun seeing where we all fit in. It was also interesting to see how correct the test was! After we took the test, we changed our office policy: all new hires would be asked to take it before the interview process began. Our doctor would then decide, based upon the results, résumé, and interviews, if a candidate was a good match for the practice.

For example, he would say, "we are looking for someone steady who is also patient and tactful." It was awesome!

There are four categories in the DISC test:

- *Dominance*—A person who is direct, result-orientated, strong-willed, and firm
- *Influence*—A person who is outgoing, enthusiastic, optimistic, high spirited, and lively
- *Steadiness*—A person who is even-tempered, accommodating, patient, humble, and tactful
- *Conscientiousness*—A person who is analytical, reserved, precise, private, and systematic

The test can be accessed online, and there is a small fee for the assessment per each employee. I've found it to be super accurate, which makes it really fun for the entire team. Find out more here: https://www.discprofile.com/

DISC helps facilitate better teamwork and teaches team members how to solve conflict when dealing with different personality makeups. It also helps you to better communicate with your patients. When you can recognize which personality type your patient is, you become a better healthcare provider. You will generally know how to prevent conflict with the patient based upon their motivations and how they are "built." You will also be more knowledgeable about how to get them to say "yes" to your recommendations.

Another test that is very popular is the Myers-Briggs Test. After someone takes this test, they'll be able to describe themselves by using a four letter identifier called a Myers-Briggs Type Indicator (MBTI), which is one of sixteen possible combinations.

The Myers-Briggs test (Fig. 19.3) breaks down like this:

- *Section one (E/I)*: are you an Extrovert or Introvert?
- *Section two (S/N)*: Are you a realistic person who likes to focus on facts? You will be classified as a Sensing person. The opposite of this would be an Intuitive person.

- *Section three (T/F)*: Are you a Thinker or a Feeler? In other words, are you more analytical or do you feel things out?
- *Section four (J/P)*: Are you someone that is a Judger, meaning you stick to plans and you are organized and prepared, or are you instead a Perceiver, and prefer to keep your options open and be flexible?

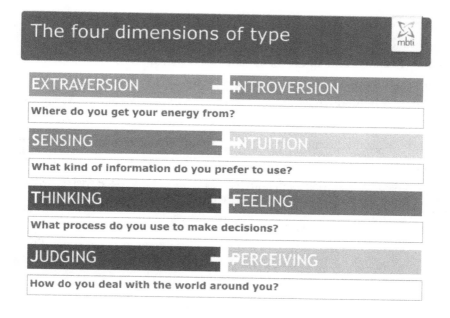

Figure 19.3 — Myers-Briggs personality types

Your combination of these types make a huge difference in how you relate to an issue and how you would possibly solve a problem. After the test is complete, and your personality type is determined, you can review your specific likes, dislikes, strengths, and weaknesses.

The MBTI is also used for team-building sessions, and as a hiring tool. It's used to analyze job applicants to determine which employees might get along with each other, and where employees will perform and fit best in the workplace.

It is super important to understand that when working with these two tests, all personality types are important. Blending them in your office should be your focus. A colorful and diverse multigenerational mix of people, from different backgrounds, including both males and females, is key to any successful business. Find the perfect mix and you'll have a recipe that can't lose.

Since this book is partly about how to make your career less stressful, you shouldn't focus solely on the day-to-day systems in your patient care, but also how calm and relaxed your work environment is. How we integrate with others through proper understanding, knowing that we're all different in our own ways, is key to office-team-work balance. We need to know where we fit and how others fit in the puzzle of productivity and social interaction. These tests promote the beginning of learning and growing as a group so that our lives continue to be enhanced in a positive way and we practice smarter and for as long as we wish to work.

Another way to make your career less stressful, and improve patient care, is finding a different way to practice—practicing with an assistant. This can be fun, for both your patient and your team.

So . . . on to the advantages of assisted hygiene!

CHAPTER 20
Assisted Hygiene: Set it Up Right and Practice with Ease

Having assistants available to us to help promote our hygiene care is an ideal way to practice. I'm sure that at least once in your career you have worked with a fantastic dental assistant who just jumped in and took X rays for you, or helped to clean and set up your room. I know when I have had this happen, I smile big and breathe easier. I really don't think that the assistants understand how much they help us. Giving us time to document our charts thoroughly, call a patient who needs to be scheduled for an appointment, or having the extra time to prepare schedules for the next day is a huge benefit to the hygiene department and to the practice.

If you are a hygienist who needs something more to fulfill your career, discuss with your doctor the possibility of starting an assisted hygiene program. I have practiced this and loved it. There have been some questions in the profession about whether assisted hygiene is a good or a bad thing. In my experience, I have seen it scheduled so amazingly, with a perfect team in place.

My first encounter with assisted hygiene was as a scheduler, before I became a dental hygienist. I was in charge of scheduling one hygienist with two scheduling columns and a registered dental assistant to help her. Those two ladies worked so well together that the patient never felt as if they were getting less of the hygienist's time. They operated as a perfect unit (Fig. 20.1). I became an instant fan after I saw the success of this. The hygiene assistant would seat the patient, go over the health history, ask the patient if they had any concerns to share with the hygienist and the doctor, and then ask permission to take the X rays. The hygienist would then enter, do the periodontal assessment and cleaning, and the assistant would jump back in and polish and floss and schedule the next appointment.

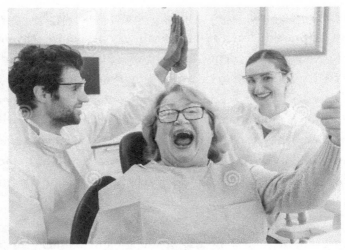

Figure 20.1 — Teamwork in action

If it worked out where the hygienist had time to polish and floss, then the two of them communicated that together and acted accordingly. The assistant was extremely gifted in directing her hygienist, telling the hygienist where to go next and what was needed. Their communication was streamlined, professional, and precise. Given that experience, I am a fan and support assisted hygiene. You just have to have the right people to run it, and it has to be scheduled well.

Most practices that use assisted hygiene schedule one column on the hour and the other column on a thirty-minute schedule. If the hygienist has an hour-long scaling and planing procedure in one column, two thirty-minute children's appointments can be scheduled in the other. The registered dental assistant can help with the children. If the kids need the hygienist's touch, then the hygienist can break away while waiting for anesthesia to take effect, or at another appropriate time, to quickly tend to the specific task in the operatory next door.

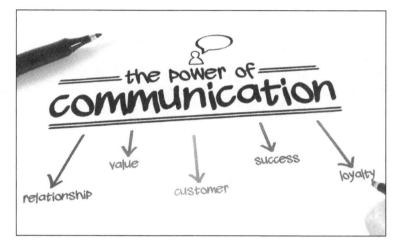

Figure 20.2 — Good communication can solve problems that crop up

Again, for all of this to be done in a timely fashion, the assistant has to be on board with the strategies of the schedule. It could be scheduled so well that a practice might have an assisted hygiene day several times a week, which also helps cut down on overhead and costs. It just depends on what you want to do in your practice, and who you have to support it. I have worked both programs, and it can be fun either way.

The good news is that with an assisted hygiene schedule in place, production can truly go through the roof! When you are seeing twelve to fourteen patients in an eight-hour day, that's an amazing volume. The art of communication (Fig. 20.2) and having efficient, hard working people in place are the key ingredients to the success of this program.

You just have to make sure that with the extra patient flow in the practice, your patients never notice the extra "moving parts" in that busier environment. The atmosphere in the practice should be stress-free and quiet. Let's face it, though: things happen. We have schedule changes, supply issues, and other situations that can throw a wrench in the well-oiled machine of our day. We have to be savvy when these situations come up, and never let the patient know when it happens.

"Remember," Mark A. Costes, DDS says, "every step in the patient experience is another opportunity to provide exceptional and memorable customer service and to distinguish you and your practice from the rest of the practitioners in your market."

So, what about the "back of the house"—how do you keep the drama offstage?

CHAPTER 21
The Back of the House: Keeping the Drama Offstage

If you are born with the gift of being able to "fake it until you make it," and can manage your moves like a chess master, then hats off to you! Some of us, as I did, had parents that were great at this skill and it rubbed off. As children, we witnessed our parents juggling two jobs, grocery shopping, and putting food on the table like it was a military operation. I grew up witnessing my mother saying things like, "We will be there in 7 minutes," and arriving on the dot. She would tell us that we would complete certain tasks "today," and that we would do it all in a given amount of time.

My mother was really great at time management and being direct in her approach when she completed a task. She never "dilly-dallied"—everything was done with a purpose. In dental hygiene, that's how we should be. We are like quarterbacks on the field, maneuvering our teammates around our opponents. Our schedules are ever changing, but we need to manage them with ease, all while winning at our game of delivering great care. We have to be confident in our approach, and once we get our systems of operation down (Fig. 21.1), we need to trust them.

It is important to systematically set up each appointment with the patient and do each step the same way, every time, keeping the same order in

175

mind and using the same phrasing to support the action. When our environment is calm and streamlined, we never appear stressed or amplified. The patient can only assume that everything is all good—even if it isn't. The patient should only see how organized we are, how high the level of care is, and how easy the appointment is for them, because our way of operating is optimum.

Figure 21.1 — A smooth-running system

"When patients are present, we are on stage," K. Pat Brown, DDS says. "The patient never needs to see what's going on backstage."

With a systematic approach to care, you will appear to the patient as if you always know what you are doing, that you are an expert. You want your patient to feel that their decision to come to you was a good one, and that they are well taken care of. Because you are operating with great confidence, they're confident the care will be excellent, and they will keep coming back (Fig. 21.2).

It's a matter of perception. The patient does not (and should not ever) know if there are potential issues in the office. As far as they are concerned, the day is filled with "rainbows and roses" and their presence with us is just the "icing on the cake."

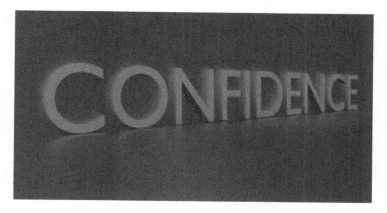

Figure 21.2 — The importance of confidence

But what if you do not have the best time management skills? In that case it is best to establish a guideline of operations for your patient's scheduled appointment time. Literally write out your approach for each type of procedure, and write down how much time is needed—even down to the minute. If the patient is scheduled for an adult prophy only, write down *all* the steps for that appointment.

An example of this could be as follows:

1. Greet patient in reception area by name and with handshake. While walking them back, ask how their day is going. Thank the patient for taking time to come in to see you.

2. Seat patient and affix napkin. Ask permission for scheduled care:

   "Mr. Smith, thank you for coming in to see us today! We have on our schedule today to clean your teeth and place fluoride to protect and prevent tooth decay. Looks like it's also time to do your images and exam as well. Is it okay if we do what is scheduled and planned today?"

Asking permission is huge! It involves your patient with their care. It makes the two of you a team, of course, and makes them feel good that you value them. So always ask permission to do everything. It also creates more perceived value because they are involved.

3. Before taking images, ask if there are any issues that they are concerned about, issues they want you to relay to the doctor (Fig. 21.3).

Figure 21.3 — Ask your patients about what's on their minds

For example, you might ask, "How is everything feeling since we last saw each other?" If they recently had a restorative appointment with the doctor, ask them how their teeth feel now that procedure is completed. Getting this information in advance helps to streamline the appointment. By gathering the necessary data, you'll make their visit more fulfilling. You don't want to find out about a toothache or other issue *after* you have already taken images and put all the equipment away. It's all in proper time management.

It is also necessary to talk as you're doing your work. We only have so much time per patient, of course, so learning the skill of talking as we complete tasks helps with our time management. We can get more done, and the flow is consistent.

The biggest skill is to operate calmly and not in a rushed manner. For the patient, it should be like watching synchronized swimmers: their feet are kicking like crazy underneath the water, but all while they appear graceful and fluid to everyone who can see the action above the water (Fig. 21.4).

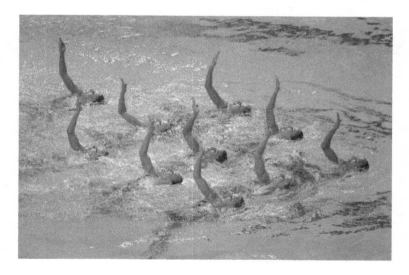

Figure 21.3 — Keeping calm, even when things go awry

This holds true if there are system breakdowns that prevent you from performing a task. When that happens, just roll with it . . . and go to Plan B. You should have a Plan B in mind for every patient, just in case a wrench is thrown into the process. The customer should never know that there are issues with the "back of the house." They should never know that something has gone wrong with your master plan.

When it does, always having an alternative action, or a "just in case plan," that will give you the peace of mind that you will get that patients' needs met to the fullest and still stay on course with your time management. Have faith! You will find a way to make it happen, and the patient will be super happy, and will never know what you had to maneuver around to meet his or her needs.

This is why you are the ultimate Hygienepreneur! No one operates like you! You're delivering the ultimate patient care.

But how do you really stay cool under pressure?

CHAPTER 22
Staying Cool Under Pressure: Never Letting a Patient See You Sweat

I have said it many times so far in this book: the Hygienepreneur's way is to stay calm in an environment that can be challenging. Hygienists are expected to do the impossible—to see every patient on time, and complete a laundry list of care, all while not rushing the visit. And we have to do it all in less than an hour, in most cases. That's a lot!

Help the patient feel like we have hours for them, even when we don't. Then, after they leave, clean your room and do it all over again for the next patient. Also, we have the doctor's schedule to consider. What if our doctor is running late for our exam? Or what if our patient who is scheduled at 10 am does not show up until 10:15 am? We are truly under the gun. Amazingly, over the years, most of the hygienists I have seen practicing next to me have been great at managing their time and making sure that the patient never "sees us sweat".

"Patients can smell fear," K. Pat Brown, DDS says. Don't let them get a whiff of it.

Our patients typically have no idea when we are running behind, or when the doctor is running behind. They have no clue that the supply order did not come in, and we are almost out of prophy paste. As hygienists, we are great at making it work and making those patients feel that during their time here in our office no issues are occurring at all, and all eyes are on them. We should make that patient feel as if they are the only patient we are seeing that day, they are number one and we value them.

But how did we learn this skill? Often it's because we had great teachers.

When we work with providers who are not good at this yet, we need to be that teacher, leading by example (Fig 22.1).

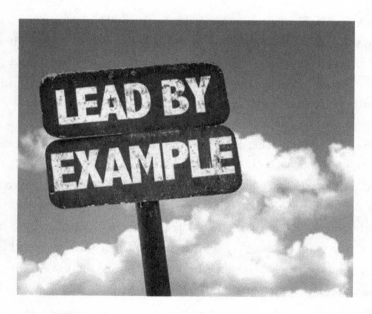

Figure 22.1 — Be a great example for your co-workers

Being a great teacher is not always about verbalizing what needs to be done. Almost always it's done by example, by showing. It's kind of like when you have a friend who you hang out with all the time, and all of a sudden both of you are using the same type of language. You rub off on each other. The same holds true for your co-workers. Not everybody is exactly the same, but when we work in close proximity with people, only hearing a certain type of language, the same way, all day long, we just naturally start to adopt it (Fig. 22.2)

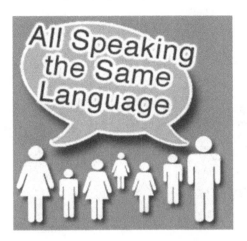

Figure 22.2 — Speak the same language as your co-workers

Being a good Hygienepreneur is being a great leader. We owe it to our patients and our practice to establish a standard of care that is above and beyond expectations. When we lead by example and show the others the systems that need to be adopted and practiced daily, we help ourselves;

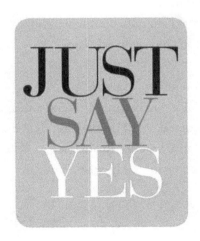

Figure 22.3 — Keeping it positive

our patients hear the same language being spoken throughout the practice. This positive and systematic culture creates a "Yes" environment. Everyone wins with this.

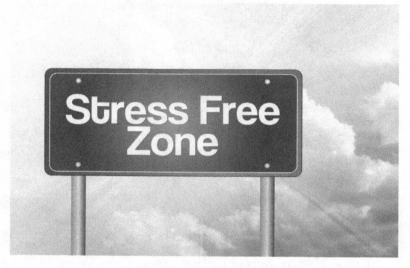

Figure 22.4 — Avoiding stress systematically

So, once you have developed a system that is successful within the practice, don't be afraid to share it. Lead, and it will rub off on the others. Again, we want to help our patients, but we also want to help our doctor to be successful. Don't lose sight of that.

No matter what situation you are facing, never show stress (Fig 22.4). Remember that you are in control of your time and of what care the patient is receiving that day. If a problem needs to be solved immediately, then solve it. Develop a "Plan B" in advance, so if the system is breaking down, another system can save the day! Being prepared is the best way to practice.

Have a hygiene meeting with your doctor and go over the systems of hygiene. Also go over the systems that solve the problems in hygiene.

That way, the end result is always good. We work in a field that is unpredictable at times. We know this, so let's take the unpredictability out of the equation and come up with answers to solve problems before they occur. Develop your system, adopt it, and practice it through role-playing. Then win! Be the provider who takes the practice to the next level! The biggest win is when your patient never knows there was an issue.

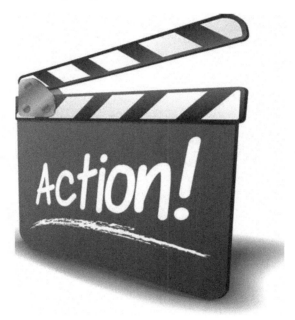

Figure 22.5 — Putting your system into practice

Now, on to Section VI, and the final frontier, focusing on *you* today, so you can continue to be a shining star for your patients tomorrow. . . .

VI. THE FINAL FRONTIER: YOU

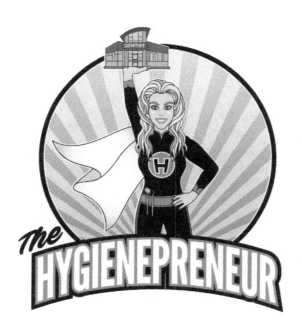

CHAPTER 23
Fitness, Wellness, and Nutrition for the Healthy Hygienist

Our jobs as hygienists are fast-paced positions that require cognitive excellence; we have to stay focused and precise, and not fail. The work can be super rewarding, but it can be very stressful if we don't manage it well. Because of this, we have to make sure that we take care of our minds and our bodies. When both are in great shape, we can endure anything. Self-care is something you should learn and practice: take time for you. Allow yourself time, and put fitness and nutrition at the forefront. Whatever it takes to start this process, make *you* a priority. Your patients and your practice will see this and thrive too. When you are fit in mind and body, these elements will spill over to your work.

At the very beginning of this book, I shared my story about my own health history. I was hustling and working two and three jobs to support my two children as a single mother, and I did not realize as a new hygienist how physically taxing the job was. During the very beginning of dental hygiene school, I remember we learned about blood pressure and health history, and we practiced gathering medical information on each other because that's what we were going to be doing for our patients before we treated them. I never considered, being so young, that I would ever experience high blood pressure myself.

Fortunately, one of the dental directors at my practice encouraged me to see my doctor. She knew that being a dental hygienist could be very intense. Managing patients and taking care of our doctors to help relieve their stresses can become physically and emotionally draining. Dentists and hygienists in school are often not given the proper tools for handling job stress. I've seen many hygienists wear the stress of their doctors and patients like a "suit of armor." They are valiant in their ability to wear it and not complain, but it's not healthy.

Reducing Stress

These emotional issues have to be addressed and managed if we're to prevent other medical conditions from erupting that could hurt our ability to practice easily and effectively. So this chapter is crucial in outlining the need to take the best care of ourselves—so we can take care of others, for a long time if we choose to.

The dental hygienists I worked with always made everything look so easy. They never seemed fatigued or stressed. Occasionally, we would hear about aches and pains, but I worked with hygienists who were a little older than me, so I attributed that information to those factors. But it wasn't so. The hygienists I was working with were seasoned professionals who'd worked full-time for many years. One practiced assisted hygiene for fifteen years and was a true professional who always showed up for work and never complained about the workload. She was the one I wanted to emulate once I became a dental hygienist. Although she had her share of aches and pains, she would frequently go to the chiropractor or massage therapist, and always show up to work the next day with a smile on her face to see our patients and take great care of them.

I thought of her when I was getting my high blood pressure diagnosis. My weight, work stress, and family history contributed to it. I knew that

I could not change my family history. However, I could make changes in the way I took care of myself through diet and exercise. I was driven to do so, because if I didn't take care of it, my career would be over. More importantly, my life expectancy would be much shorter.

Controlling Your Weight

In my initial years as a dental hygienist, I battled weight. I would lose and gain weight like crazy. My focus was on working and building dental practices and providing for my children, not on my health. Thankfully, one day I woke up and I was just "sick and tired of being sick and tired."

As I've written earlier, I started the journey to weight loss through .surgery. During the weight loss adventure, I also hired a personal trainer who discovered that my core muscles were extremely weak. The trainer focused on abdominal strength in order to help prevent back pain in the future. As dental hygienists, whole body health is very important: if we are physically healthy, it will improve our mental health ,which in turn helps reduce stress.

I wish I'd learned that before I started, but in hygiene school there was no class on how to take care of ourselves so that we could have a long life of practice. Financial management classes were not offered either. And, of course, no personal physical fitness courses! All of these areas are important to know about, because any one of them can be a dealbreaker when it comes to being the best provider we can be.

Throughout this book, I've talked about being a Hygienepreneur, which means being in charge of your "practice within the practice." That means covering all aspects of the job. Remember, it is not just about delivering great patient care and succeeding financially, it is also about taking care of yourself and winning.

Fitness and Nutrition

There are two basic formulas for taking care of your body as a dental hygienist: proper nutrition and physical fitness.

In an article published February 14, 2014, *RDH Magazine* listed dental healthcare professionals as the second highest risk category out of 974 occupations for exposure to colds and flu, mainly because we sit and practice in such close proximity to our patients for long periods of time. As hygienists, of course, we must practice close to our patients, and we must deal with the oral cavity, a place where bacteria thrive. Taking the proper nutritional precautions to increase sustainability is important. Naturally, we should build up our immune system to combat this risk. I am not a medical doctor, but there's a lot of anecdotal evidence to suggest that supplements can help. Talk to your doctor about what will work best for you, based on your specific needs and your system. Proper nutrition will help you fight any of the bugs that are out there and reduce your risk of getting sick. Also, don't forget to get proper rest. The body needs sleep to refresh and repair itself. When we are not resting, our bodies can't get ready for the next day of work.

Along with proper nutrition, physical fitness is a huge aspect of being a high performing dental hygienist. Most dental hygienists I know work to maintain good physical fitness. I've seen many of them doing different workouts that promote abdominal core strength to properly support the spine in order to prevent injuries in the back and neck, and the stress they bring. Everything is connected. Good health starts with a strong core.

Strong abdominal muscles protect the back and are the foundation of core strength. Weak core muscles can result in a loss of adequate lumbar curve and poor posture, an imbalance that can lead to upper back pain, lower back pain, and neck pain. Good core strengthening exercises may include planks, bilateral leg raises, and traditional sit ups. Practicing good posture helps keep the core stable too. A strong abdominal core and good nutrition will help us practice pain free.

Certain equipment we use in our jobs can also help. Wearing "loupes" or magnification glasses helps our posture by helping us sit right. If we lean or bend the wrong way when using these devices, our view of the oral cavity and the tooth we are focusing on can become blurry. Again, discussing the best way to achieve your personal success with your health and fitness provider is where it should start.

Nutrition Tips

Make it a priority to discuss your nutrition and diet with a nutritionist or a medical provider who you trust and who knows you. My medical provider recommended the following supplements for me:

- *Vitamin D*—Its benefits include supporting muscle function, bone health, and immune function.
- *Zinc*—My doctor said zinc was the most important supplement of all because so many people are deficient in zinc in their diet. It aids in immune system health.
- *Vitamin C*—A very popular supplement, Vitamin C is known to protect the body against infection.
- *Super Lysine*—This supplement is known to increase calcium absorption, which can reduce diabetes-related illnesses and improve gut health.
- *Elderberry*—It has long been used to treat infections, is high in antioxidants, and is known to also help lessen inflammation and reduce stress.

Along with oral supplements, good eating habits are also important. It was recommended to me to eat more vegetables like carrots, sweet potatoes, kale, collard greens and spinach. These are naturally high in vitamins and minerals. Also, we have to go back to the basic information we all heard in our middle school nutrition class: eating fresh fruit helps combat disease and infection. Fruits that are high in antioxidants and phytonutrients include blueberries, bananas, and mangoes. These helpful foods are sometimes forgotten about as we get into the hustle of our working lives after we finish hygiene school. You have to remember to take care of yourself so you can continue practicing in the profession that you worked so hard to join.

As we've discussed, being healthier systemically and financially is a core attribute to becoming a Hygienepreneur, but we also have to have the courage to be honest with ourselves and consider whether we truly are doing everything to better ourselves. I had to look in the mirror and say to myself, "Am I doing enough?" Was I just going through the motions as a practitioner, or was I going to move into the next phase in my career? I had to give myself a pep talk, and a dose of reality. I became physically healthier and, in the process, became a driver at my dental practice.

But what next? We were soaring and my doctor was happy because the practice was successful and the patients were happy. So, it was time to have "the talk."

CHAPTER 24
Have Courage! Talking to Your Boss About Your Future and Your Goals

Fact: 60-75 percent of all dentistry revenue comes out of the hygiene department.

When we have goals, we must write them down with timelines so the possibilities that these will be attained increase. Every year, usually at the start, my doctor and I sit down and establish what my goals are for the next season in my life. They used to be about physical health and internal office career goals and productivity. Now, because I continue to hit those marks, I've chosen something different.

In 2018, I sat down with my doctor and told him I wanted to write a book. He said, "how can I help you?" This was huge, to have a boss who was supportive of my goals both in and out of the office! Whatever your goals are, have the confidence and faith to sit down with your doctor and let him know. Ask for his guidance and help as your employer. You never know what ideas and support you can obtain with the meeting.

Most hygienists are not comfortable with the business side of hygiene; it's often not something they've studied, or feel they are "built for." But understanding the "yes" helps to overcome those internal conflicts. Doctors need to involve their staff with the numbers and not keep the practice's business hidden. That way, the staff is more comfortable about decisions that help not just the patient, but the business as well.

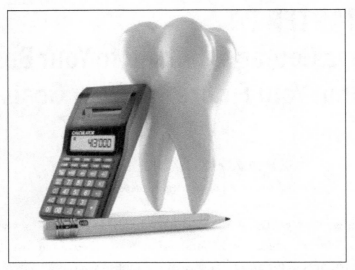

Figure 24.1 — Dental health and financial health

When the staff knows that the practice is financially healthy, they will feel more secure about their jobs and will work with more confidence. It is always such a great feeling to have an employer that you know is going to take care of you and has the means to do so. We all know that when the practice is doing well, there are more benefits available to the staff. The results of success definitely trickle down. We must realize that when the business is doing well, it enables us to open the doors to tomorrow, and to provide more services for our community. It really is a win-win for everybody.

As K. Pat Brown, DDS says, "When you have the solution, the conversation will be easy."

As producers, hygienists need to understand what the practice overhead costs are and what the hourly goals should be to meet those overhead costs (Fig. 24.2). We need to help our doctors achieve their goals. When the dentist achieves success, big things can happen for the dental staff: benefits and salaries can increase. We need to make sure, as loyal staff members, that we focus on the financial health of the practice first.

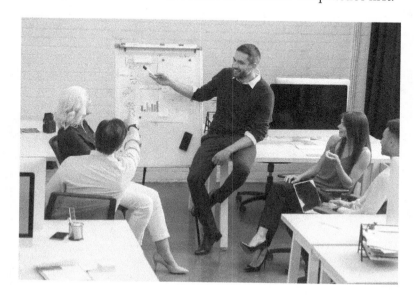

Figure 24.2 — Keeping everyone informed

If we see that the practice is doing well and that our position has produced growth, then it makes sense for a hygienist to be able to sit down with her doctor and talk about extra perks. Some hygienists will operate on a fair hourly wage and negotiate a bonus based upon goals being met.

According to Mark A. Costes, DDS, a wise dentist recognizes that sharing success has many benefits:

> *You're investing in your own financial freedom when you set proper salary levels and proper bonus levels for every member of your team. When your net income increases as radically as that of all of your staff, you won't mind those few extra dollars in bonus money that you are paying out. You'll come to realize that the*

more dollars you pay in bonuses, the more thousands of dollars accrue to your own personal bottom line.

Other hygienists will be satisfied with the financial terms of a fair hourly wage. Whatever works for your practice, your doctor and you, is good (Fig. 24.3).

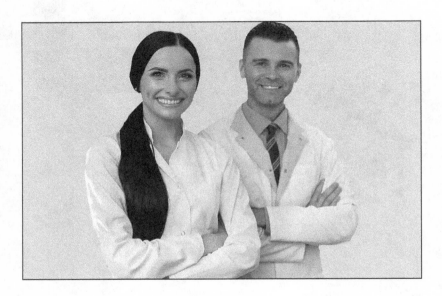

Figure 24.3 — Sharing in the success of your practice's team

Believe me, the hygienists who I have trained have told me that as Hygienepreneurs they are all getting paid more money because they are working more productively and with less stress. Their doctors appreciate the difference in their work attitudes compared to other hygienists, and the pay scale recognizes that. It is important for our hygiene culture to convey a sense of compassion, confidence, intelligence and grit. We can do anything, and we can take our careers to any level that we want. We respect our field, respect the dentists we work with, and we want to see their practice success elevate, reaching goal after goal.

To be the best we can be, we have to add creativity, knowledge and savvy practice management to our practices. If we do this, the hygiene culture at our practices will be positive and motivating. Leading by example, a hygienpreneur's passion for patients and the practice is invaluable and necessary to withstand times of uncertainty. We demonstrate how to rise above any challenge, like superheroes ready to save the situation on any given day. Becoming a Hygienepreneur is a genius move, one that fills in the big picture of gaining the financial security that we once could only dream of. Let's be smart: work hard, start now, and you will see this kind of success.

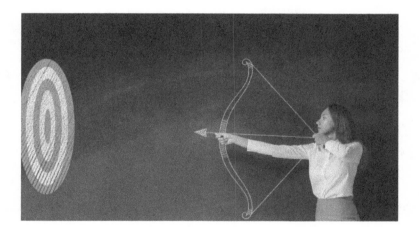

Figure 24.4 — Targeting success

But what about finding personal financial tranquility? Let's dive in . . . .

CHAPTER 25
Finding Financial Tranquility

Maintaining a fantastic career is one of the most crucial components of becoming a true Hygienepreneur, it's not just about working hard, it's about working smart. We have to learn early to save for a rainy day in order to practice and grow tomorrow. As a single mother of two, I learned this lesson very late. But I learned it!

I feel that it is important to include this final chapter in the book because it is the most critical one when it comes to maintaining "whole health." It's not just about office health, patient health, and physical health. You have to make sure that you have great financial health. I learned from both of my parents that even if you are a married person, you can't always rely on your mate and their income.

It was 2004, and I had just had a major water leak at my home. There was a crack in the slab: pipes had broken and that led to some major damage. After all the leaks in the pipes were fixed, there was rehabilitation that needed to be done to the house. The plan was to place new drywall, new flooring, new carpet upstairs, and of course paint and baseboards to get everything back to the way it was. I was on a break from dental hygiene school and my dad suggested that he and I could do the work together to save money. This would also allow us to use better quality materials on the house than the builders had used. It would be a ton of work, but I knew the payoff would be huge.

The demolition began and I worked side-by-side with my dad, tearing up flooring and learning how to prep tile and put wood flooring in place. I tried to protect my hands while doing all the tasks, but I ended up going back to hygiene school with cuts and bruises all over them. It was, however, worth it!

Initially, I thought it was worth it because of the money it saved, and because I would have better materials and upgraded products in my house. But later I learned that it had been worth it because it gave me that one-on-one time with my dad, time that I later recognized as being so valuable.

As we worked on my house, I noticed that he was suffering from fatigue I had never seen before in him. My dad was a workhorse, an executive chef who always worked three different projects as well as helping everybody, someone who never said *no* to anyone. He gave back to charities by cooking thousands of meals, all while working at multiple jobs and maintaining his own company.

When we were using the tool to lift and cut up the flooring, he kept asking me to take over, joking that I wasn't doing my part. Later, though, I would realize that his body was suffering from a disease that caused weakness in his extremities—amyotrophic lateral sclerosis (ALS), also known as Lou Gehrig's disease.

My dad was diagnosed in 2005 with ALS, which would claim his life less than one year later. It was terribly rough on my family. My mother stood by him until the end, taking care of him and just trying to keep him comfortable. She has always been an example for me, a loving and educated professional woman. She has always worked extremely hard, just like my dad.

During that time, I saw her rise to a whole other level as both caretaker and provider. For many years, my mother had been Director of Nutrition at Valley Center Unified School District. Thankfully, she did not have to drive very far to work every day. But I saw her go back and forth between work and home to help my dad. He went from using a cane to using a walker, to being in a wheelchair, and then to being totally bed bound in less than eleven months. He passed away on November 21, 2006.

The emotional and physical strength that my mom showed during that time was so impressive to me, as was the way she handled the finances. To this day, I still do not know how she did it. But, I learned at that moment that it would be very important, whether I was to be remarried or not, that I needed to be financially self-sufficient.

Becoming Self Sufficient

I cannot stress this enough! As a hygienist, trying to make your way, this is one of the most important chapters in this book. If you're a young hygienist, right out of school, learn these tools now. If you're a seasoned hygienist, like me, it's not too late to make the changes necessary to reach your financial retirement goals. The key is to start. Today!

About six years ago, one of my more persistent friends wrangled ten of us together to go to Dave Ramsey's "Financial Peace" course. My eyes opened wide in the first class. His courses focus on things like investment strategies, saving for a rainy day, saving for the long term, and becoming debt-free really quickly. I began to practice his formula right away. Long ago I'd made an important decision: I'd bought a house, which I worked hard to keep all the years when I was a single mom. It taught me a big lesson: be sure to pay yourself first, so you are taking care of "later."

As hygienists, and Hygienepreneurs, our jobs are physically and mentally difficult. However, being a hygienist is also a very rewarding career. The financial stability that can come from it has led it to be rated as one of the top professions in America to consider. They did not teach a retirement or "financial game plan" course at dental hygiene school, but I was lucky enough to have an instructor who recommended a great book, *The Richest Man in Babylon*, by George S. Clason. It's a quick read, and it will open your eyes to the possibilities of financial success. Start reading it now!

There are many ways to become financially self-sufficient, but remember that things happen in life: people get divorced, spouses become disabled, spouses can even pass away, as my dad did. More commonly, a spouse can suffer from a job loss. All this is to say that we need to make sure that our one income can "carry the house," both today and tomorrow.

The principles in this book talk about how to increase patient care, improve practice health and, in turn, help yourself become more successful. But knowing how to handle that success is critical too.

Basic Financial Smarts

I am not an expert on financial planning, but I am an expert at making mistakes, learning from them, and making the changes necessary to succeed. So, if you have a friend or family member who can help you with this, just do it. Please, don't wait. I don't have any regrets, and I am proud of the fact that I began this mission wholeheartedly seven years ago. I have not looked back.

Along the way I've listen to those who are experts to help me take the guesswork out of this area. After all, this is my hard-earned money, and I have to protect it and make it grow. I often mention what I learned from Dave Ramsey because of the courses I took years back that helped me.

One of the areas he covers is the "Steps to Financial Peace." These include the following:

1. Make a money plan.
2. Change the way you do things.
3. Manage your money.
4. Name where your money should go.
5. Be frugal and money savvy.
6. Strive to be debt free.
7. Don't charge or borrow—only buy what you can afford.
8. Pay off debt.
9. Invest in the future.

Making a plan for your money is important. If we know how much money we make each paycheck, and "tell it where it's going to go," that helps us to make sure that all of our goals are being met. We had a plan on how to get into hygiene school. We need to make a plan on how our money will be directed and placed. We need to be proactive with our money. We need to figure out what we want to do with it and make this our reality. When we do this, it will *become* a reality!

Once you've made a plan and listed the goals for your financial future, and what you want your money to do, you need to make changes to increase the chances that this will happen. It takes discipline to grow as a person. You may have done this already in other areas like diet and exercise. Financial health is just one more area that you need to dig into and put in the effort and be consistent with. Recognizing the plan and putting in the work to make changes will ensure that you have more money to direct to your future. Learn to say "no." Learn to not impulse buy. Learn to research a purchase and get the best price. We are adults, not children, and we need to act like it. You will be empowered by nearly instant results!

You have to start doing things differently if you want a different result, Dave Ramsey says: "Twelve-steppers say if you continue to do the same thing over and over again and expect a different result, that's the definition of insanity. You have to change the path."

Financial Tools

Learning to manage your money is truly a life skill I did not learn while growing up. My parents were hustling and didn't have the time to sit and discuss it, but it's a very important life lesson. Some high schools are teaching this now; I truly applaud their efforts in offering this important skill to our youth.

But as usual, I had to learn the hard way that moving forward and doing it now is what is important. So, again: "Tell your money where you want it to go." Write it down. Whether you ask a financial planner for help, or go to a class, get a notebook and make it your financial workbook, the place where you can write your goals down and then live by them. Reference it, and keep it active.

There are many software tools and financial systems that help you manage your money. Having auto-deposit enabled in your personal checking account, where funds are allocated to separate accounts, is a common way to pay bills. My budget categories are *Groceries, Gas, Medicine/Pharmacy, Hair care/Makeup, Car Maintenance, Personal, Entertainment and Gifts*. If you use budget-tracking software, it is important to give every dollar a location before the month begins. Operate on a zero-based budget, where all money is allocated before being spent. This ensures that your budget is being maintained and helps make sure *you* are being paid too.

Dave Ramsey puts it this way: "You must gain control over your money or the lack of it will forever control you." It's so true! Give every dollar an identifier. It should be allocated and named. Creating a budget and allocating specific funds to certain things will keep you on track. Whether you're paying off debt or paying house bills for the family, every dollar needs to be counted.

"You're making every dollar behave," Dave Ramsey says, "giving every dollar a name before the month begins."

Start a budget by figuring out what your total income is. Then list all expenses—from the regular bills to the small incidentals. Make an attempt to adjust the expenses until they are equal or less than your income. This can be a fun game! Tracking your expenses month to month, and then adjusting your spending behavior, will ensure better money management. You'll be controlling your money, not letting it control you.

Know What You Can Afford

Be frugal and money-savvy today so you can have wealth tomorrow. I had to learn early on not to feel the need to "keep up" with the other baseball and softball parents when my children were playing sports. They had money, low debt, and dual incomes. I was living paycheck to paycheck, on one income, but I did learn some survival skills that carried me through until I really learned good money saving principles. Hygienists, please strive not to be "dual income dependent" if you have a significant other. As I mentioned earlier, things happen in life. It is always best to live as if you only have one income. Everything else is extra. By keeping our spending within our income and only buying what we can afford, we create a positive environment where our money is now ready to work for us.

Dave Ramsey's measure for whether you can afford something is simple: If you can say, "'I wrote a check and paid for it," then you can afford it. "That's the definition," Ramsey says. "If you can't pay for it in cash, in total, on the spot, cash on the barrelhead, you can't afford it — whatever it is, your car, your clothes, your groceries."

Paying off debt allows more for savings tomorrow. I learned how to pay off small balances first, while still making minimum payments on the large ones. Then I could concentrate on the big ones. Once the money I'd allocated for the small balances was paid off, I could roll it into payments on the big ones as well. It had a domino effect, and worked fast. I felt good about it, which made me want to do more.

Again, there are many methods of attack. Find what works for you, but recognize that it needs to happen, and follow through with the plan. Invest in your future: you do not know how it will turn out! You need to be proactive.

If your office offers a 401k plan, sign up for it and maximize your contribution—especially if there's an employer match. You won't miss the money. Once your balances are paid off and you are not adding debt, and your budget is working, then you can decide how much and where to start investing beyond what's possible with your work plan. To be in this position is huge. As a Hygienepreneur, who is successful in and outside of your practice, your confidence and happiness will show through to your patients and those who work with you. Though, again, I'm no financial expert, I nevertheless pride myself in listening to people who are, following a plan, and growing professionally and personally!

In Closing...

To be the best hygienists that we can be—to be Hygienepreneurs—means to add creativity, knowledge and savvy practice management to our work. If we do this, the culture at our offices will be positive and motivating. Leading by example, a hygienpreneur's passion for patients and the practice becomes invaluable and necessary in times of personal and professional uncertainty. We rise above any challenge like superheroes, ready to save the situation on any given day.

Your license gives you not only the right to call yourself a professional hygienist, it's also the ticket to win and succeed every time. Savor it like one of the printed golden tickets in the *Willy Wonka and the Chocolate Factory* movie! Know the value it holds, not just for a successful dental practice, but as a source of confidence and success for your life!

Now, go forth and be part of the new movement. Spread joy and success, and be the Hygienepreneur I know you can be!

For more information on training pathways, visit my website:
THEHYGIENEPRENEUR.COM

APPENDICES

APPENDIX 1
Dental Hygiene Scripts

Training the office with scripting is crucial to the success of your practice's case acceptance. When your patients understand the treatment that is recommended and everyone explains it in the same way, that builds confidence throughout the whole practice.

Scripting conversations between team members and patients is a valuable tool that everyone will benefit from. Listed below are some of the general scripts for a dental hygiene department. Once the team learns a script, they can put their own flair on it so the message will sound more natural and flow easily. Case acceptance will increase throughout the practice, and patient health will benefit too.

Many times in meetings with my team, I practice scripting, and even utilize the extra tool of videotaping myself and my team members so we can see what our body language looks like when we are delivering our message. Earlier in my career I found myself pausing a lot, or I would use certain words repeatedly. You never really know how you will be perceived until you see yourself on video. Honestly, it's super awkward in the beginning to watch, but it becomes kind of fun after you start doing it, like a game. And it's really fun for the team to play this game together.

In all seriousness, though, it really is valuable; it makes your job easier. You find yourself not having to think so much to answer patient questions, which reduces stress and promotes ease of practice. So go for it and you will see the results! As K. Pat Brown, DDS says, "If you have ever said something that didn't come out the way you intended, you understand the value of a script."

Front Office

You may wonder why you need to know phone scripts that are usually for front office personnel. During down time, you should be on the phones, and will find yourself experiencing these situations. With these skills, you will become an asset instead of a burden during down time. You will benefit by filling your own schedule as well.

Answering the phone

Say it with a smile!

FRONT OFFICE: "Thank you for calling Dr. Jones's office, this is Wendy. How may I assist you?"

Confirming appointments

FRONT OFFICE   "Hello Mr. Smith! This is Wendy from Dr. Jones's office. How are you doing today?

Great! I'm calling because we look forward to seeing you for your reserved hygiene/doctor appointment scheduled tomorrow Wednesday, April 15 at 8 a.m. We will see you then! Have a great day!"

Note: When leaving a message, say roughly the same thing.

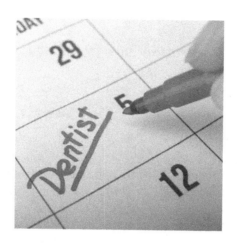

Scheduling hygiene/doctor appointment

FRONT OFFICE: "Hi Mr. Smith! It's so great to hear from you today! May I help you?

Of course we can schedule you a doctor/hygiene appointment. Do you prefer a.m. or p.m.?"

Note: Only provide two choices.

Patient appointment–Asking to hold for scheduling coordinator

FRONT OFFICE: "Hello Mr. Smith, it's great to hear from you! How are you doing today? What can I do for you?

Mr. Smith, I am sure we can accommodate you and get you taken care of. Our person in charge of scheduling is a whiz at finding a convenient appointment time for you. Would you mind if I place you on hold briefly so I can inform her of your needs?

Great! She will be right with you. Thank you so much."

Note: Inform the scheduling coordinator of the patient's name and a detailed reason for their calling to schedule.

COORDINATOR: "Hello Mr. Smith. I understand that you need an appointment for *[the doctor / hygiene]* Let's get you taken care of."

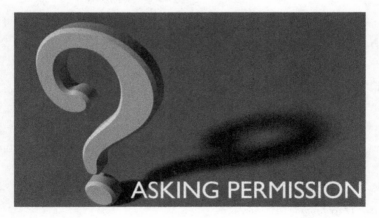

Note: When you must place patients on hold, always ask permission first, and thank them when you reconnect.

Reactivation call

FRONT OFFICE: "Hello Mr. Smith! This is Wendy from Dr. Jones's office! How are you?

Great! How is your family?

We were calling today to check in with you to see how you're all doing and schedule your hygiene appointments. Did you know it's been a year since we last saw all of you?

We have missed you and have been thinking of you and thought that we would give you a call. What days are best for you to come in?

Would you prefer morning or afternoon?"

Note: Only provide two choices.

Rescheduling missed/canceled appointments

FRONT OFFICE: "Hello Mr. Smith! This is Wendy from Dr. Jones's office. How are you doing today?

Great! I was calling because we missed you for your [doctor / hygiene] appointment. We wanted to first make sure you and the family are *okay?*

Oh, that's good to hear. So what days work best for you?

Morning or afternoon?"

Note: Only provide two choices.

Same-day cancellations

FRONT OFFICE: "Hello Mr. Smith! It's great to hear from you! We look forward to seeing you later today for your reserved *[doctor / hygiene]* appointment.

Oh, you are not able to make it in today? I hope everything's *okay?*

Is there any way that you could somehow still come in today? Maybe we can make it work in another way? We reserve time for only you and the [doctor / hygienist], and it is difficult to offer the appointment to another patient with this short notice."

Note: If the patient says no, unless you have availability tomorrow and are desperate to fill it, be sure to act. It's good to "seem surprised" that you do have a last-minute unexpected change for tomorrow and offer it to them. Always remind your patients how very busy the schedule is. We always want patients to keep their appointments and not to cancel!

FRONT OFFICE: "Mr. Smith, we understand that sometimes things come up that are out of your control. Let's get you rescheduled for a day that will be better for you. Oh, I'm surprised. Looks like we have an unexpected change for tomorrow at 10 a.m., would you like to reserve that time?

Okay, great! We look forward to seeing you tomorrow, Tuesday, May 21 at 10 a.m. Have a great day!"

Unscheduled treatment

FRONT OFFICE: "Hello, Mr. Smith, this is Wendy from Dr. Jones's office. How are you doing today?

I was calling to check in with you. The last time you were in our office, the doctor recommended that tooth number three on the upper right side was in need of care. There was deep decay present under an existing large amalgam filling and the tooth was in need of a crown. I researched your insurance plan and it looks like they will pay approximately 50% of the fee. So your portion due that day would be 400. *Okay?*

Great! Dr Jones has availability for you Monday, June 3rd at 3 p.m., how does that sound?

Great! Your fee that day will be 400. Mr. Smith, again we look forward to seeing you Monday, June 3rd at 3 p.m. Have a great day!"

Note: *Don't say "400 dollars."*

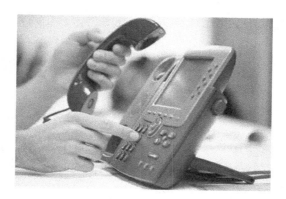

Why do I need a hygiene appointment in three months?

FRONT OFFICE: "Mr. Smith, our hygienist recommends that you come in every three months to help manage the condition. According to the Board of Periodontology, bacteria re-colonizes every ninety days. This is the bacteria that invaded the infection or gums and caused the destruction of gum tissue and bone. With your history of gum disease, it is very important that we clean below the gum line every ninety days to remove debris and eradicate the bacteria that is present. This will help ensure that your condition will not get worse. We get fabulous results when patients follow the schedule and follow through with their home care."

New patient experience initial appointment call

Note: Answer within three rings.

FRONT OFFICE   "Thank you for calling Dr. Jones's office, this is Wendy. How may I help you?

That's fantastic, who am I speaking with?

Jon, when was the last time we saw you?"

He says he is a new patient.

"That is great, Jon! We are so happy to hear from you! May I ask you a few questions so we can get a time reserved for you?

Great! Let's get you taken care of soon. It looks like we just had an unexpected change for a cleaning appointment tomorrow with our hygienist, [*hygienist's name*]. She is caring and gentle. It is at 10 a.m. tomorrow. Would you like to reserve that time?"

He says that he can't come in tomorrow.

"*Okay*, no problem. What days are good for you?"

He says that he is off work on Mondays.

"*Okay*, that's a great day to have off, Jon! Do you prefer morning or afternoon?"

He says that he likes mornings.

"I have next Friday, September 4th at 10 a.m. available for you!"

He says that is perfect.

"I am so glad. The appointment is scheduled with [*hygienist's name*]. She is so caring, gentle and thorough; she's going to take great care of you! Along with your cleaning, is it *okay* if we complete images and have the doctor complete a full exam for you?

He agrees.

May I do anything else for you?

He says no.

> "We look forward to seeing you next Friday. Have a great rest of the day."

Hygiene Department

Hygiene greeting new patient in reception

Greeting new patients in the reception area like you would at the front door of your own home is key to making them feel comfortable. That five-star customer service shows through when we display the extra touches. It is critical to do what others aren't doing, to greet people like they matter and that you appreciate them. Let's face it, there are dental offices out there on every corner, but this patient has chosen you. It is *okay* to treat the patient with gratitude and appreciation for doing so.

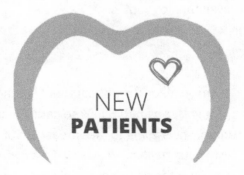

Walk out to where the patient is seated and address the patient by name:

HYGIENIST: "Hi, Randy. Welcome to the practice. My name is Shalon. I am one of Dr. Jacobs's hygienists. We are so happy that you are joining us today! Would you mind following me? We are going to take great care of you!"

Note: When patients are leaving after their appointment is done, thank them for choosing you and your practice. Tell them that you appreciate them for making the choice and trusting you with their dental health.

LBR (Laser Bacterial Reduction) adjunct

While measuring the patients gums, let them know that you are going to measure the space in between their teeth and gums.

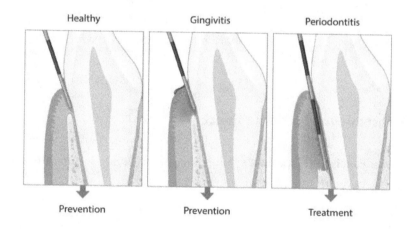

Healthy	Gingivitis	Periodontitis
Prevention	Prevention	Treatment

HYGIENIST: "Twos and 3s are healthy numbers, 4s mean gingivitis. If it's 5 or above, we will talk about it."

Note: After completing the perio assessment, sit the patient up. Here is an example of how that conversation can go:

HYGIENIST: "Mrs. Smith, we have completed your perio exam. What we are seeing today are areas of inflammation and signs of gum disease. You have 4 and 5 mm pockets with bleeding. The areas are specific to your molars and premolars. In order for us to help preserve your bone, we will need to treat the areas in a special way. What we will do is clean the areas thoroughly, removing all the tartar buildup and plaque, then we'll disinfect and reduce the bacteria that is under the gumline using a laser. With its laser energy it will reduce the bacteria count from millions to hundreds. You won't feel it, which is awesome. Then we will see you every three months to maintain these areas. Then we just have to make sure that you brush, floss, and use your waterpik every day. The fee for the laser is $49, and I will treat your entire mouth. Can we go ahead and take care of that for you today?"

LD (Laser Degranulation) adjunct

While measuring the patient's gums, say you are going to measure the space in between the teeth and gums:

HYGIENIST: "Twos and 3s are healthy numbers, 4s mean gingi-vitis, and 5 or above we will talk about."

Note: After completing the perio assessment, sit the patient up. Here is an example of how that conversation can go:

HYGIENIST: "Mrs. Smith, we have completed your perio exam. What we are seeing today are areas of inflamma-tion and signs of gum disease. You have

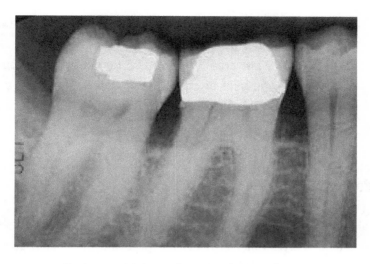

Patients with bone loss need special care.

4 and 5 mm pockets with bleeding. The areas
are specific to your molars and premolars. You
have a few areas where the tissue is extremely
infected. In order for us to help preserve your
bone, the doctor recommends we treat the areas
in a special way. What we do is clean the areas
thoroughly, mechanically removing all the tartar
buildup and plaque, then we disinfect and reduce
the bacteria that is under the gumline using a
laser. We will also be using the laser to remove
diseased tissue from inside the pocket. With its
laser energy, the laser reduces the bacteria count
from millions to hundreds, and by removing the
infected tissue this will help the tissue to shrink
and reattach to the root, giving the tooth healthy
support. You will be comfortable while we are
treating the areas. We will numb the areas so you
will not feel a thing. Then we will need to see you
every three months to maintain these areas. We

just have to make sure that you brush, floss, and
use your waterpik every day. The fee for the laser
is 49 per area, totaling 196 for your entire mouth.
Do you have any questions? Can we go ahead and
take care of that for you today?"

Initial scaling and root planing

It is always part of the hygienist job to continue to explain and go over the
patient's treatment plan after the doctor completes the periodontal diagnosis
and shares his procedure recommendations and then leaves the operatory.
The patient will look to us to help guide them and assure them that they are
making the right decisions about their dental health. We are truly their part-
ners in this process. Because we are their periodontal experts, it is important
for us to have all the answers when it comes to the periodontal procedures
that are available to them to help preserve bone and gum. The scaling and
root planing procedure is important in preventing future surgical options.
We need to get the scripting right so that the patient will follow through with
the care and understand the value and results that it will produce.

HYGIENIST: "Mrs. Smith, after reviewing your periodontal
assessment, the doctor recommends that you
have a special procedure completed to help
improve your periodontal health. This procedure
is specific to treat the gum and bone in a special
way. It is called scaling and root planing. This
procedure is amazing because it not only allows
us to gently remove debris that is stuck deep in
the pockets on the roots but it also allows for the
removal of diseased gum tissue that is present
in the pockets. This is a nonsurgical approach

to the treatment and maintenance of periodontal disease. You will be comfortable during the
procedure. We usually treat half the mouth at a
time with special numbing agents. Again, you will
be comfortable in the process. Afterward, we will
see you for a follow-up appointment to check to
make sure that the inflammation of the gums has
reduced and that the gums respond in a positive way. After that, we will see you every three
months to make sure that the bone and gums
stay well maintained and that your homecare
supports this process as well."

Why do I need a hygiene appointment in three months?

HYGIENIST: "Well, according to the Board of Periodontology,
bacteria re-colonizes every ninety days. These
bacteria invade the areas and cause destruction
to bone and gum tissue. With your history of gum
disease, it is very important that we clean below
the gum line every ninety days to remove debris
and eradicate the bacteria that is present. This will
help ensure that your condition will not get worse.
We get fabulous results when patients follow the
schedule and follow through with their home care."

Scaling and root planing (existing patient)

Sometimes it is necessary every two to three years to do either
complete root planing (code 4341) or limited root planing (code 4342)

in areas to help maintain periodontal health. When this is necessary, a special message needs to be delivered to your patients letting them know it is time to move forward to do this. It depends what you and your doctor see and conclude. At one of the periodontal recall exam visits, your doctor can discuss this need with your patient. If it has been two to three years, and an area seems like it needs root planing, and/or the gum tissue inside the pocket requires inadvertent curettage, your doctor can inform your patient of the need and then you can schedule this accordingly. You will be giving a great service to your patient to help them prevent future periodontal surgery, and you will be actively boosting your production within your schedule. When we do the right thing for our patient and are proactive, everyone wins. The message from your doctor can be delivered like this:

DENTIST: "Ms. Rita, you and Kelsey have been doing such a great job maintaining your gum health. However, there are a few areas that are in need of special root smoothing and planing again. Every few years it may be necessary to gently go under the gumline to smooth the roots of debris and roughness, and while doing so also remove diseased tissue so that healthy tissue can attach to the roots again. I feel that it is time to do this to help continue the process of maintaining good periodontal health. Kelsey is going to continue being your partner in this, and whenever the two of you can coordinate your schedules to complete this, that would be great!"

Note: After your doctor leaves, you can piggyback off of what he said and then do it that day if you have time, or schedule a time that is good for the both of you. Even if it is very limited (code 4342), it is still good to help promote healthy gum and bone, and to reestablish that they are indeed an active periodontal patient.

Adult fluoride adjunct

Our society has long accepted that fluoride is recommended and given to children who come into our dental practices. The American Dental Association has also long recommended topical fluoride treatments for adults who are at high risk of decay.

Some factors that increase a patient's risk of developing caries are drug or alcohol use, active caries, poor oral hygiene, eating disorders, lack of regular dental care, poor diet, existing restorations, tooth enamel defects, and decreases of salivary flow (medication risks). There are a few others that we all know about, but this has been a widespread issue that dental professionals have had to realize and inform our patients about regularly. It is a serious cause for concern, one that has left us educating our patients about the recommendations and benefits of topical fluoride for our adult patients.

One of the challenges that I have heard is that insurance does not cover the adjunct treatment. I recommend that you nevertheless establish a fair and reasonable fee for those patients who do not have the coverage and always offer it. The script can be as follows:

HYGIENIST: "Mrs. Jones, I am so happy that you are here today and that we were able to complete your periodontal assessment and continue to establish that we are doing a great job in maintaining your periodontal health. You are using good tools at home and are coming in regularly, which is great. My only other suggestion is something that Dr. Sam discussed with me—the addition of in-office fluoride to your visits to help prevent recurrent caries. You have a lot of existing restorations with margins that plaque is sticking to. We want to make sure on those vulnerable areas that demineralization does not occur, resulting in a cavity. Protecting these areas is so important! Also, during my gum assessment I documented all of your recession areas. Root exposure can lead to root cavities. Your enamel is like granite, but your roots are like sandstone. Plaque can stick to the roots more easily because of this. Decay can start on a root that is not protected. It would be good if, after your dental cleanings, we placed fluoride varnish all around your existing restorations and root surfaces to help prevent tooth decay. It is sticky and the tooth absorbs it well, like a sponge. Your insurance does not cover it, but we offer a special fee of only 26, as we can to do it at the end of each of your hygiene appointments. It will be awesome to help maintain everything. Okay?"

Note: *Do not say "dollars."*

Cervitec Plus by Ivoclar Vivadent adjunct

Another challenge is patients who worry about the effects of fluoride on their systems, and do not want any in their bodies. In the past, when patients responded that they did not want fluoride in their body, we would say that it was okay in moderation. We would share studies that showed there was no danger in small quantities being used every 3-6 months. Nowadays, patients do not want to hear this information. Our society has access to more health knowledge than ever, so they often have already made up their minds about what is good for their bodies and cannot be swayed. It is better to offer an alternative that works so that they see that we are respecting their beliefs for their bodies, all while meeting our goals of protecting and preventing. So offer an alternative and get the "yes. Remove the potential struggle and both of you win.

If your patient refuses fluoride for systemic and dietary reasons, you need another option of prevention. Cervitec Plus is great for the gums and helps fight tooth decay. It can be placed all around the margins of restorations and on root surfaces very easily, like fluoride, for the patient who refuses fluoride. This product contains chlorhexidine and thymol, and controls bacteria. It is clear in color and generally can be applied every three months to protect teeth, root surfaces, hypersensitive teeth, and tooth surfaces with active bacteria, and works spot on.

HYGIENIST: "Mr. Grable, it is great that you are coming in regularly, and your mouth is under a great maintenance schedule. The doctor is concerned about protecting what you have. Your existing restorations and root surfaces are at a higher risk for recurrent decay and this is always a concern. As you know, we are all about prevention. We would definitely recommend fluoride after your hygiene appointments to help maintain these areas and protect your investment. We want your existing dentistry to stay clean and healthy."

Mr. Grable says he does not want fluoride, ever.

"I understand your apprehension about fluoride. We do know that fluoride used in moderation has a lot of benefits to help prevent tooth decay. But it is even better that we now have an alternative to fluoride available for you that not only helps prevent tooth decay but also helps the gum health as well. It has chlorhexidine and thymol in it, is completely safe, and has no fluoride. The doctor has made this available to us for patients who do not want fluoride, or who are allergic to fluoride. So, it will aid in the prevention of recurrent decay around your existing dentistry and protect your root surfaces as well. The fee is only 26, and it is completed at the end of your visit like fluoride. Afterwards we ask that you don't eat or drink for just one hour. Okay?"

Note: *Do not say "dollars."*

Arestin adjunct (Code D4381)

Along with scaling and root planing, Arestin is a common and effective procedure that we will suggest to help treat and maintain periodontal conditions. An antibiotic agent, it aids in the suppression of pathogenic bacteria and is designed to remain inside 5+mm pockets long enough to provide therapeutic benefits. Sometimes we have patients who need it after scaling and root planing when we are checking them at their first periodontal exam. If there is a need for further treatment, this medicine can be placed. There may or may not be a fee to the patient if insurance is involved. It is great when we are able to know in advance what patient insurance will cover and what the fee may be if this procedure is necessary. Remember, we are always fighting with time: if we know that this is our patient's first periodontal exam after root planing, or we have evaluated our patient's history before a standard three-month recall periomaintenacne appointment, then we can determine the possible needs in advance. Finding out the fee in advance so that we can quickly quote it ourselves saves time from asking and waiting for our front office to deliver the message.

This adjunct is very important for patients' health and can leave your patients happy and satisfied, knowing that they are being offered the best care available. For us, time is of the essence, so get the information in advance and take control of your schedule. Present the fee and treat the area with ease.

HYGIENIST: "Mrs. Turner, after completing your periodontal assessment today, I noticed that the healing response from the completion of the scaling and root planing that we did has been great. I am very pleased with the results. I am sure that you are feeling better as well? Your hygiene care has increased as well in all of these special areas, which also is very helpful for maintenance. However, while I was checking the areas, there were still a few pocket probing depths where the numbers were higher, and that are still inflamed. These areas are more advanced in the progression of the disease and require a little more help. The doctor recommends we place antibiotics in the pocket to help reduce the pathogens that are causing the continued infection. It is safe and extremely effective for areas just like these. As long as you are not pregnant or nursing or allergic to Minocycline or Tetracycline, we can use this procedure to help prevent surgery in the future. There are three areas that need it and your fee is 50 for each. Your total due would be 200. I will

place it at the end of your appointment today
after the areas are nice and clean. For seven
days after, do not eat any hard, sticky, or crunchy
foods. Do not floss, pick, or waterpik the area for
ten days. Okay?"

Note: Do not say "dollars."

Night guards

If your doctor has previously recommended a night guard, and the
patient still has not had the procedure completed, gently suggesting
that it's still needed will help your patient a lot. This is also an opportunity to increase your hygiene production with just a quick impression.
Reminding and helping your patient to be proactive about completing
this care is of great value. You will be assisting them in protecting their
bone, gums, and tooth structure. In the morning, after reviewing your
schedule, you should look out for this procedure so that you are prepared
to offer it if need be. If the procedure has not yet been diagnosed by your
doctor, but you are reading that there are signs of need, you can easily
ask your doctor to evaluate tooth wear and make the suggestion. Ask
your front office what the patient fee is, in advance if possible, so that
you can present it and deliver the care quickly and efficiently.

HYGIENIST: "Mr. Smith, I see that all of your restorative care
has been completed. Great job on getting every-
thing completed! How do you feel?

I did notice that the last need that you and doctor
planned was to protect all your new dentistry,
bone, and gums with an appliance that you will
wear at night called a night guard. This guard is

crucial in aiding in the protection of your teeth, dental work, bone, and gum tissue from the grinding and clenching that you do. Your fee for this is 400. I can easily take the impression today for you. You can schedule a follow-up in a week for the delivery of the appliance. Okay?"

Note: Do not say "dollars."

Whitening adjunct

Patients want whiter teeth. You will be amazed how many are ready to start the process once you mention it. Take the time to discuss it and you will give your patients the ticket to a whiter and brighter smile that will make them so happy. Also, this is a great way to increase your daily hygiene production. It is easy and fast to complete. In less than ten minutes you can increase revenue for your practice, and your patients will thank you for helping them. If you are a hygienist who is able to perform in-office whitening in your chair, you will see even bigger rewards. Promote the procedure and have fun with it.

HYGIENIST: "Mrs. Lacky, your gums and bone levels are looking awesome! It is so great that you are maintaining yourself so well. If you wanted to whiten your teeth, this is a great time to do so. We have several options to make this happen for you. We can take impressions for you at any time and give you a custom kit that you use at home. We also have the ability to reserve time, about two hours, and whiten you here in the practice. It is easy and very relaxing, and the results are fantastic. We have seen some of our patients getting up to

234   APPENDIX 1

eight shades lighter! Included with the fee ,we
make you trays to take home, and give you several
tubes of the whitening gel for you to maintain
your whiter smile at home. Either procedure is
super effective. For the take-home trays and kit
alone, the fee is 350. The in-office whitening with
the maintenance trays are 600. We can do it for
you whenever your wish."

Note: Do not say "dollars."

Your patients will then tell you if they are interested. If they are, enter
it in their treatment plans. Let them know you have time today to take
impressions for the whitening that costs 350. If they want to reserve the
time with you for the in-office whitening procedure, reserve it in your
schedule when it is convenient.

Adult sealants

This procedure is of huge benefit to your patients. What a great service to
offer! Adult patients are easy to treat. If needed, the procedure is usually
completed on one to two teeth, and should take less than ten minutes. If
the tooth has stain present, you will want to use a perio sand polisher, or
ask your doctor to very quickly clean out the groove with a burr. It requires
no anesthetic. Have the high-speed handpiece and burrs ready there when
your doctor is completing the exam. You can ask the doctor in front of
the patient if the tooth would benefit with a sealant placement to prevent
tooth decay. Having everything available will ensure that your doctor can
jump in and clean out the stain very quickly, with no time wasted. You can
pre-inform your patient as well of the fee, and let them know you want
to confirm with the doctor that the tooth will benefit from this procedure.

HYGIENIST: "Maggie, your molar on the upper right has stain present deep in the grooves that put it at an increased risk for tooth decay. If the doctor thinks it is necessary, we can clean out the groove and place a sealant in the tooth to prevent this from happening. When the doctor comes in to do your exam, I will have him check it, *okay?* If he thinks we should do it, the fee is only 35, and will take less than ten minutes. Let's check with him first. If the two of you agree, I can do that for you today with no problem. *Okay?"*

Child sealants

This is a well-known procedure that is of great service to all children. Review your schedule in the morning and note whether there are any children scheduled who still need sealants. Ask your front office about insurance benefits and tooth history, so when the opportunity presents itself you are ready to complete this procedure on the same day, with no time wasted. Know the benefits and fees in advance so you can inform the parents and get the yes with ease. Always be prepared! Also, ask your front office if there is coverage if a sealant needs replacing. Sometimes, if a sealant was placed a long time ago, sealing may need to be completed again. Knowing all the information in advance will help you deliver the care, all while being on time for your next patient. Same-day performed sealants are a great way to increase hygiene production, all while delivering super care.

HYGIENIST: "Mr. McDonald, I just cleaned Jeremy's teeth, and the doctor completed his exam. Great news! He is still part of the no-cavity club. The doctor wants to make sure that Jeremy stays cavity free, and it is time to place sealants on his permanent molars. This is a great way to prevent tooth decay, and it will only take me less than fifteen minutes. We want to go ahead and get the teeth protected today because they are all clean and ready. The girls in the front already said that your insurance will cover this procedure for Jeremy at 100%. We are good to go. Okay?"

APPENDIX 2
Interviews with Three Successful Dental Hygienists

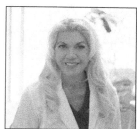 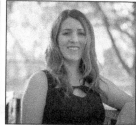 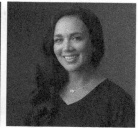

(L–R) Tiffany Cavazos, Shalon Ziegenhorn, Cortney Dickert

Personally, I am a hygienist who takes pride in the fact that I did not just graduate from hygiene school and work for one doctor forever. I graduated, and then started to work temporary assignments at many practices. I served as a temporary hygienist all over Southern California. I filled in at all different types of offices. Some focused on families with children, while others had clients that strictly served older folks, with no children. I even worked at specialty practices, for top periodontists, which taught me so much.

My goal was to see where I would fit best. I wanted to practice where I felt comfortable and would flourish. During this journey, the offices I worked at were of all different sizes, and had different dentists with different mission statements. And, of course, they all took different types of insurance plans.

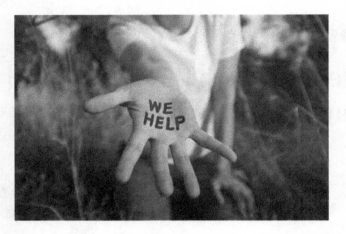

Hygienists were born to serve others.

These offices were also located in different socioeconomic areas, so they charged different fees for their services. The caseloads ranged from easy to advanced, based on the areas where I worked. I was not shy about treating the more advanced cases. I loved helping people of all walks of life manage their oral health.

Even if I was only there for one day, I was on a mission to deliver the best care, no matter what I was getting paid and no matter where I was working.

Even today, I still occasionally temp to keep my skills sharp and to gain different perspectives on how other practices manage their offices. I like to add to my skills and up my game, and to bring tidbits of information back to my home base that my teammates and doctors might possibly adopt.

Recently, I collaborated, side by side, with amazing hygienists from different practices, Shalon Z., of Menifee, CA, and Cortney D., of Hendersonville, TN. I talked to them about their perspectives on where the hygiene field is going, and what the daily challenges are that hold them back from winning every day.

Together we discussed common questions that we all continue to hear from our colleagues and our peers, so we thought we'd see how, together, we could solve some issues that regularly occur in our field. Here are some of the questions we discussed, and our answers.

Question: Staying on time

I cannot seem to stay on time with my patients' appointments. What are some techniques that I can adopt that will help with my time management?

Answers:

SHALON:
"Adopt a routine. I find it helpful to start in the same area on every appointment and work my way through the entire dentition until done. It also helps to review charts at the beginning of the day and make sure procedures are loaded into the schedule to avoid any surprises (like FMX, sealants, etc.)"

CORTNEY:
"Organization is the key. I try to review charts before the patients arrive so I know exactly what I am doing that day. I also make sure I have trays stocked, water filled, and supplies ready to go before the day starts to help with time management."

TIFFANY:
"When I come into work in the morning I 'prep' my day. I look at possible treatment needs that

are not scheduled. I make sure that my schedule is accurate. Are all the necessary treatment needs on the schedule? Are X rays and an exam needed? I also look to see who my patients are that day and if they need special care that requires more time. If they need an exam, and they're a patient who likes to talk, I will alert the doctor in the morning so we can practice good time management together. I might even move the patient to another room for their exam, so if they want to take more time with the doctor, I can still see my next patient on time."

Question: Ensuring future appointments

How do I make sure that every patient leaves with a hygiene appointment? The patient always says they do not know what they will be doing in three or six months.

Answers:

SHALON: "During the hygiene appointment, I usually ask what a good day and time is for their next appointment, that way I can schedule them before they leave. Sometimes you get the patient that doesn't know what their schedule will be like down the road so I always say, "we will just go ahead and get you on the books so we can keep track of when you are due and if you need to change the appointment or move it to a different day, that is perfectly fine." Patient acceptance is pretty high after I explain that to them."

CORTNEY: "Do not give them the option to not schedule. Avoid saying, 'Can I schedule your next appointment?' Rather, say, 'Let's schedule your next appointment.'"

TIFFANY: "I say to them, 'let's go ahead and schedule your next appointment.' When the hygienist schedules it, patients are more likely to say yes. Plus, I can schedule for exactly how much time I will need and even preschedule the proper procedures that I will do that day. Because I am the one seeing them, the appointment is scheduled more accurately. If a patient says that they do not know what their schedule is like in three or six months, I tell them, 'let's go ahead and get it scheduled so that way you have your reserved time. You will get a reminder text two weeks before the appointment and if you need to make a change, that is when you can do that. We just get so booked up, so I want to make sure that you have your time reserved.'"

Question: Refusing fluoride

What do you tell patients who refuse fluoride? They might mention that the media says it is dangerous. What verbiage can I use to convince them of the benefits versus the risks?

Answers:

SHALON: "I explain that many years of research has been done on the benefits of fluoride and it has been proven that fluoride reduces caries rate, reduces tooth sensitivity, protects existing dentistry, and remineralizes the tooth."

CORTNEY: "I don't argue with them. I let them know that the harm they are talking about is when fluoride is taken in large quantities. I tell them that I respect their beliefs and that I want to make sure that I share the need to help prevent caries."

TIFFANY: "When they refuse fluoride treatment, I give them another option, Cervitec Plus, which benefits the patient against demineralization, sensitivity and helps fight gum disease. If you give the patient an alternative, it reduces their concerns and you get the yes!"

Question: Insurance denials for SRP

Insurance companies keep denying scaling and root planing (SRP) in patients with obvious clinical disease. How can I increase my chances of insurance companies approving the proper therapy my patients need?

Answers:

SHALON: "Some great options to increase the acceptance of SRP from an insurance company would be submitting intraoral photos and possibly vertical bitewings (instead of horizontal, because they show better angles of the bone loss). Also, noting in the patient's chart where the bone loss is present and what surfaces have radiographic calculus is a good idea."

CORTNEY: "Make sure you have a current full-mouth radiographic exam, current pocket probing depths recorded, with bleeding noted, and a narrative."

TIFFANY: "In order for insurance companies to pay for SRP with obvious signs of periodontal disease, it sometimes may not be enough to just submit radiographs and probing depths. Another way to get insurance companies to cover the procedure is to let them know if the patient has any comorbidities that hinder their ability to heal. For example, diabetic patients are a huge risk for periodontal disease."

Question: Avoiding chaos

Exams are a chaotic mess in my office. How do I keep the doctor and myself on task and streamlined to save time?

Answers:

SHALON: "When the doctor enters the hygiene room, always be prepared with radiographs up on the screen so you can discuss any complaints the patient might have along with your findings. I write down what areas I have found with possible decay or fractures or areas of inflammation for him to examine without having to study every single tooth since I have more time with the patient than the doctor does."

CORTNEY: "A morning huddle and a good assistant to guide the doctor on where he needs to be does the trick for us. We also use headsets to communicate, and they work really well."

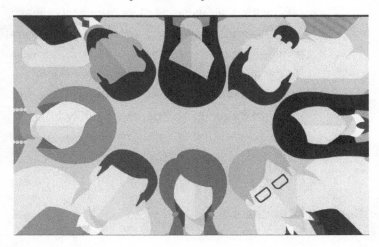

TIFFANY: "First, we practice, practice, practice. What I mean is that we role play and script every step of what happens during a new patient exam and the existing patient exam. They are both a little differ-ent. Once we jot down what needs to happen, step by step, then we are prepped and ready for the patient. We have even video taped ourselves during the roleplaying process to hear and see what works and what doesn't. I prep my schedule every morning and then I let my doctor know what is coming ahead. I give him the entire story and then we go through our hand off system and it is quick and streamlined. It is very organized. Every exam we do uses the same format and is carried out in the same manner. It just works!"

Question: Someone needing a lot of work

I have a new patient who has not been seen by a dentist for 25 years. He has received prophies every 6 months. He has obvious signs of periodontal disease, bone loss, and tissue loss. What's the best way to approach this patient without overwhelming him?

Answers:

SHALON: "The best way to approach these patients is by educating them on what we are seeing. It is a great idea to take intraoral photos along with a full mouth series of images, and put the findings on the TV screen or the computer, and visually show them where their bone height should be. Then, go over the probing depths with them and explain the findings in a way that is easily understood. I always explain that a prophy is for a patient that has no bone loss, no signs of gum disease, and healthy teeth and gums. Each patient is different and some may take more time for acceptance of SRP, and a three-month recall instead of a six-month recall. For the patients who are absolutely against SRP and/or a three-month recall, I usually say, 'We can re-evaluate these areas on your next cleaning.'"

CORTNEY: "Tell him what you see today. I always verbally (out loud) complete the periodontal assessment. In the beginning, I inform the patient that I am checking to make sure their bone and gum support is healthy, [and tell them] they are going to hear lots of numbers, and that three and below are good numbers. When patients start to hear me say fives and sixes, they typically ask me what that means, and that is my opening to patient education. I also show X rays with bone loss, and take intraoral photos to show calculus."

TIFFANY: "I have had this happen so many times! I have temped in other offices and experienced this. I will typically do my assessment and say that there has been evidence of the destruction of bone. I inform the patient of the degree of bone loss and then I say, 'It looks like inflammation and bone loss was seen on your last images and periodontal readings. We were trying to see if increased hygiene care would reduce inflammation, but it just hasn't. We may need to take a different approach.' Then I bring the doctor in so he is involved, and we decide on a plan together with the patient. We are the patient's advocate. When they see that we are there to guide and help them, but that they are in charge, case acceptance is achieved."

Question: Another hygienist's problem patient

A patient who is new to me has been seen in the practice for the past ten years by another hygienist. They have been receiving six-month prophies. They have obvious signs of bone loss and tissue loss, red bleedings gums, and 5 mm pockets. The Patient refuses SRP. How do I best approach this patient?

Answers:

SHALON: "It is difficult to have patient compliance when they have been seeing another hygienist for ten years, SRP has never been recommended in the past and most of the time periodontal disease has not been discussed. The best way to approach these patients is by educating them and explaining your findings and then recommending whatever the best treatment is for that particular patient. I give them the information that is needed and it is ultimately up to the patient to make the final decision."

TIFFANY: "I educate the patient and let them know that I couldn't sleep at night unless I told them what was going on. I would also get the doctor to see if his words would help to get 'the Yes.'"

CORTNEY: "This is a difficult question, and one I have experienced many times. I let the patient know that we are seeing evidence of bone loss and gum disease. I say that our approach is not working and we need to modify the plan so we can protect the current bone level."

Question: Encouraging referrals

My patient literally kisses the ground I walk on. They sing our praises when they are here. How do I turn this patient into a "practice builder"?

Answers:

SHALON: "We will ask the patient to give us a video testimonial. We let them know how nice it will be for new patients to hear a critique about our office from an actual patient. They almost always say yes. They like us and want to help us. And we appreciate it!"

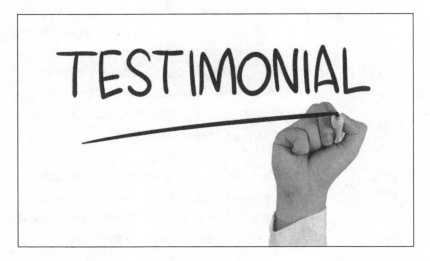

CORTNEY: "If the patient already sings your praises, then that is a practice builder, right? We give every patient referral cards in their home-care bags. If a patient says how happy they are, I always ask if they wouldn't mind leaving a review on Google."

TIFFANY: "I immediately say thank you so much! I tell them the reason we do what we do is because of patients like them. I ask if we could please get a picture with the doctor, and if they would mind doing a video testimonial. A lot of times patients think that our practice is not accepting new patients, but we always do. We just have to ask them to refer their friends and family. We want to treat other nice people who are just like them. They love that!"

Question: Front office issues

My front office lacks the motivation to support the hygienists in the office. I find myself calling to confirm patients, preparing financial arrangements, and constantly asking them to fill my schedule. How do I appease my front office and get them to do what I need so the practice flourishes?

Answers:

SHALON: "The best way to approach these type of situations would be to directly talk to the dentist/owner of the practice and have him address the issues with the front office. I sometimes feel that if I complain to the front office, they are not going to take me seriously or want to help me confirm my schedule and fill it."

CORTNEY: "It starts from the top, down. The doctor needs to be clear on protocol and what is expected of the front desk."

TIFFANY: "I come at it from a different angle because I used to work in the front office earlier in my career, and I know how overwhelming that job can be. So I approach the front and petition their help, and ask them how we, as a team, can solve the issues of appointments not getting confirmed or financial arrangements not being completed. I ask them what their system is to fill the schedule, and say if I have downtime I can help, but, 'Is there anything that you can do to solve the issue? Because I know that you are experts at it.' I try to approach them with positivity and understanding so I can get my needs met. Then, if I still see an issue, I will approach the doctor and ask him to help with solving the problem. The person in charge of a certain task may just need some training. Sometimes accountability trackers can be utilized to help with the success of filling the schedule. The accountability trackers are usually tracked by the manager or the doctor, so that he can see that everybody is doing their very best to keep the schedules filled."

Question: Shaky handoffs

Handoffs between my doctor and me are shaky at best. How do we improve our presentation and verbiage?

Answers:

SHALON: "Every office should have a protocol for what verbiage should be used with every patient at every appointment. If we explain our findings and have the necessary information ready for the doctor when he or she arrives, the handoff should go smoothly for each patient and most importantly, be consistent."

CORTNEY: "Have a script. And use it!"

TIFFANY: "Handoffs to the doctor are super important. It helps us communicate everything important that we need to communicate. It also helps us keep ourselves on time so we are not communicating things that are unnecessary. We focus on what is necessary and deliver the message in a precise manner that both the doctor and patient can understand. It needs to be decided in advance what information is important to the doctor and what is important for the patient to hear from the doctor. Then each hygienist needs to prac‑ tice hitting those points every time. The practice sessions can happen during a monthly meeting, where each hygienist branches off and practices handoffs with the staff and the doctor. The team can see what works and what doesn't, and modify it before seeing a patient. Then we utilize that system for every patient, the same way, every time."

Question: Improving front office answers

My front office is answering hygiene questions and not succeeding with the patient. How do we all get on the same page in regards to using the same verbiage across all staff so that we are all fluid and we "get the yes"?

Answers:

SHALON: "Communication is the key. Having monthly or weekly meetings with the staff can increase the chances that everyone is on the same page."

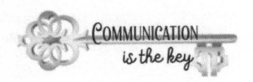

Answers:

CORTNEY: "There is a technique called 'questions in a hat' that we have used and discussed in our office meetings. We all drop questions in a bowl that patients have asked us. Then we, as a group, answer them and agree on how we will respond to this question if a patient asks us. That way, we all are answering it the same way. The patient will hear the same answer no matter who they ask."

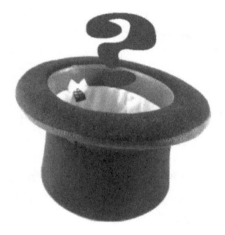

TIFFANY: "Our doctor has told us how he wants us to answer certain questions. And all of us answer the question the same way, every time. If we find that these questions continue to come up from our patients, then we sit down as a team and figure out how we need to change our answers so that way the patient will understand better."

Question: Getting patients to understand

My patients never seem to retain what I explain to them in detail. What methods can I use to make sure my patients understand what their needs are and accept the recommendations we have given them?

Answers:

SHALON: "Using visual aids probably works best. You can use your computer screen and or TV to put up radiographs and intraoral photos to show areas of concern or even areas of their mouth that look great."

CORTNEY: "I like to use pictures that the patient can see. I use their photos and show them healthy areas and non-healthy areas. I also give them literature to take home and read. We also use YouTube a lot to explain procedures. We have found certain YouTube channels that we like and always refer to those. It really helps."

TIFFANY: "We love to use YouTube dental videos. We first show them their pictures and readings, and then show them the videos that match their condition and needs. We definitely make sure the videos are short and sweet. It is such a great aid."

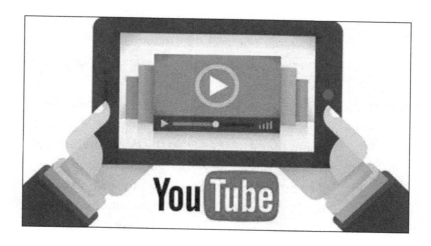

Question: Keeping patients committed

I have a high success rate with SRP case acceptance, but it seems like a lot of patients don't stay committed to consistent perio-maintenance. How do I make sure patients are educated so that they stay consistent?

Answers:

SHALON: "Educating patients is the key to success. In our office we perio chart at every hygiene appointment and are constantly discussing bone height, increase and decrease in probing depths and areas of bleeding and inflammation. If patients are aware of their periodontal status and want to refrain from losing teeth and bone, then they will be compliant with regular perio maintenance."

CORTNEY: "It needs to be made clear from the beginning of patient education that 'once perio, always perio.'

Also, the facts should be discussed. Let them know that bacteria reformulates every ninety days and that you can provide evidence if needed."

TIFFANY: "Once a patient has SRP, they need extra care to maintain the current level of bone. I stress to them that if we can keep the bone where it's at right now then we will be good for a long time. The bacteria that contributed to their disease is evident and still active. I share with them relevant studies and that we know beyond a shadow of a doubt that a three month schedule of good perio maintenance cleaning with good home care are the two things that can keep their disease stable. The disease is always present. With good care by both parties, the disease can stay dormant and nonaggressive. They usually understand after we take the time to really explain it to them."

Question: How to fill schedule holes

My schedule looks like "swiss cheese"; lots of holes in it! How can I ensure that this doesn't happen consistently?

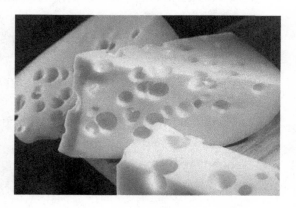

Answers:

SHALON: "Making sure front office staff is all on the same page helps. If the office has protocols on filling the schedule and they stick to it, then there shouldn't be holes on a consistent basis. Making sure patients are being reminded the day or two before the appointment seems to be the key. If an appointment is made six months in advance, patients have to be reminded or they will forget and there will be holes in the schedule".

CORTNEY: "Patient education, so they value their appointments and see the importance. If a patient cancels, do not reschedule them right away."

TIFFANY "We keep a list of patients that are ready to be scheduled on a short call list. When patients try to reschedule, we tell them in a polite manner, "are you sure that you can't make your appointment today? Our schedule is so booked and I'm afraid our next opening for you will be several weeks out." This trains the patients to know that appointment times are valuable; that it is not an option to get another appointment right away. If they still reschedule, we push them out and ask if they want to be added to a short call list if, by chance, another appointment pops up.

Question: Getting an assistant

I approached my doctor about assisted hygiene. My doctor says we can't afford another assistant. How can I justify and explain that I will be more productive with the aid of an assistant?

Answers:

SHALON: "Assisted hygiene has the potential of making double, even triple the amount of production compared to non-assisted hygiene. There are pros and cons to both, it just depends on the type of practice the doctor wants to run."

CORTNEY   "Showing the doctor that assisted hygiene mimics how the doctor practices is a way to integrate familiarity. Everyone is doing their part and it makes the schedule more streamlined and, at the end of the day, more productive. The patient feels like they are more cared for because there are more people interacting with them during their appointment."

TIFFANY   "It really takes a complete synergistic operating system and team to support assisted hygiene. Everyone needs to be on the same page and all goals and communication has to be 'on point.' Once that is established, then it works well. The doctors don't usually need too much convincing if it is run well with no headaches, the patients are happy, and we're showing good margins."

Question: Keeping things interesting

I feel like every day is like the movie "Groundhog's Day", where it's a repeat of the previous day. How do you maintain an excitement and energy when your job can seem so routine?

Answers:

SHALON: "Being passionate about my career and caring about my patients helps to keep me motivated and excited to go to work. For me, every patient has a story and everyone is different, which keeps the day from being routine."

CORTNEY: "Embrace all we can do with hygiene; prophylaxis, perio TX, sealants, laser . . . the list goes on. It's hard to get on board with variation. Also, I always get excited when I go to local hygiene group meetings!"

TIFFANY: "I engage with my patients. I have fun with them. Listening to all of their life changes and growth is so interesting. Then when I have down time I live life! I get outside, travel and rest. Keeping my body healthy is also important to me. It is so important to stay fit. It helps with your job performance and job enjoyment."

Wrapping Up

Looking over these common issues and coming up with resolutions to the questions has helped us in our daily routines at my office. We reduce stress and operate at a higher level when we can move past the issues that seem to repeat themselves across our industry. Sometimes, we need to get together and figure out a common thread that will enable us to deal with an issue and move forward so it is not continuing to hinder our "fun" at work.

Remember, we are trying to reduce a common problem in dental hygiene: early burn out. Our profession has been compared to that of stockbrokers. We "turn and burn" all day long. If we don't find ways to reduce our stress and to practice with ease, we could be part of a statistic. Hygiene students will be facing the same issues when they go out into the world of dentistry and I want to help prevent their stress level from being so high. I want to save them years of frustration early on so they can enjoy our great field and become productive Hygienepreneurs early in their careers! If I knew then what I know now, I would have saved myself years of frustration and of fighting for the "golden ticket." I'm still learning every day. But now, when I learn, I have a strong foundation, and it is super motivating to be able to build upon that and "get the win" with a great deal of satisfaction.

Mike Czubiak, DDS and Steve Sperry put it really well: "Traditional thinking will kill today's dental industry. If dentistry is to survive and improve patients' health, then creative leaders, dentists, hygienists and teams must change. Did you know that nothing grows in ice? If we let tradition 'freeze' our minds, new ideas can't sprout."

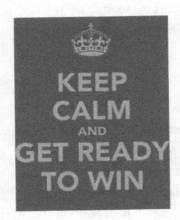

Index